Table of contents

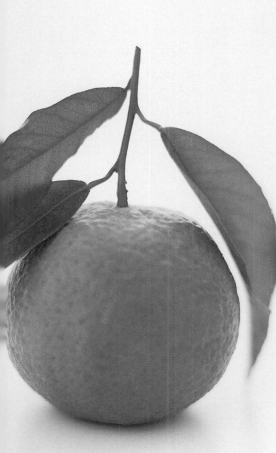

616
.1205 MAYO-C   2012h

Mayo Clinic healthy heart
for life!

P9-EAY-409

YOUR BIGGEST RISK	**8**
Warning signs of heart disease	11
Common myths about heart disease	12
Risk factors for heart disease	14
PART 1 ~ GET GOING!	**16**
CHAPTER 1 Get ready to start	**18**
Do you need to see a doctor?	20
Are you ready to start?	22
CHAPTER 2 Eat 5, Move 10, Sleep 8	**24**
Take a baseline quiz	26
Work on your goals	27
PART 2 ~ 10 STEPS TO HEART HEALTH	**32**
Making the Mayo Clinic Healthy Heart Plan work for you	**34**
CHAPTER 3 Eat healthy	**36**
Boost your vegetables and fruits	38
Eat breakfast ... and eat it right	39
Go for the grains	40
Focus on fats	41
Be lean with protein	42
CHAPTER 4 Be active	**46**
Stand up for heart health	48
Start with 10	48
Add intervals	50
Boost your strength	52
Pick things you enjoy	52
CHAPTER 5 Sleep well	**56**
Aim for consistent quality sleep every night	58
Get adequate sleep to help you lose weight	59
Establish a consistent bedtime routine	60
Be cautious about caffeine and alcohol	61
Make sure you don't have a sleep disorder	61

Table of contents (continued)

CHAPTER 6 Deal with tobacco and weight   64

Tobacco and heart health   66

Weight and heart health   68

CHAPTER 7 Know your numbers   72

Blood pressure   74

Cholesterol   74

Triglycerides   77

Body mass index   78

Blood sugar   78

CHAPTER 8 Know your history   82

Personal history   83

Women's unique risks   85

Family history   85

CHAPTER 9 Set your targets   90

Your personal risk   92

Plans to reach your targets   95

CHAPTER 10 Take your medications   98

Understanding the problem   100

Overcoming the challenges   102

Side effects and interactions   104

CHAPTER 11 Plan for emergencies   106

Recognize the warning signs   108

Delay is deadly   109

Start CPR if someone's in trouble   110

Use defibrillation, if necessary   112

Involve your family   113

CHAPTER 12 Enjoy life   114

Build a social support network   116

Relax and have fun   117

Reduce stress   118

Learn to be adaptable   120

Find a realistic balance   121

Using the Mayo Clinic Healthy Heart Plan for a lifetime   122

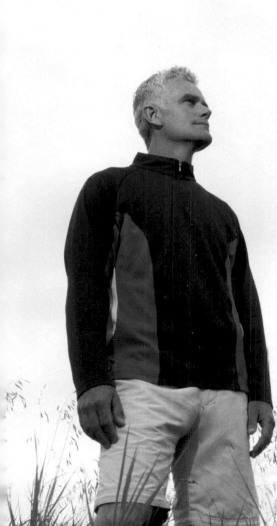

PART 3 ~ IF YOU HAVE A PROBLEM   124

CHAPTER 13 How your heart works   126

CHAPTER 14 What can go wrong   136

CHAPTER 15 Coronary artery disease   144

CHAPTER 16 Heart failure   156

CHAPTER 17 Arrhythmias   166

CHAPTER 18 Heart valve disorders   176

CHAPTER 19 Vascular disorders   186

CHAPTER 20 Congenital heart disease   196

PART 4 ~ HOW TO SUPPORT YOUR PLAN   206

CHAPTER 21 Common diagnostic tests   208

Blood tests   209

Electrocardiogram   210

Stress tests   211

Imaging tests   213

Taking your blood pressure   216

CHAPTER 22 Overcome your eating obstacles   220

Recipes for a healthy heart   234

CHAPTER 23 Overcome your activity obstacles   244

CHAPTER 24 Find a healthy weight   254

What's your BMI?   257

The Mayo Clinic Healthy Weight Pyramid   259

CHAPTER 25 Complementary and alternative medicine   260

Common herbal and dietary supplements   262

Food as medicine   264

Mind-body medicine   266

CHAPTER 26 Monitor your mental health   268

Stress and your heart   269

Recognizing depression   273

Taking care of anxiety   275

Index   278

Forward

You may use expressions such as "my heart is broken" or give someone "heartfelt thanks," but are you aware of what the heart is doing every minute of your life? Your heart pumps 2,000 gallons of blood through your body every day. Given the complex and vital function of this organ, it's not surprising that things can and sometimes do go wrong.

Heart disease affects all of us, either directly or indirectly. It is the leading cause of death in the United States. You may feel bombarded with conflicting information about heart health: What's good, what's bad, and what do you really need to know? That's the reason we've written this book — to provide a clear program to help you have a healthy heart for life.

The good news is that most heart disease is preventable. And keeping your heart healthy doesn't require a lot of time and effort. Small changes, such as standing up and moving more, can make a big difference. The changes don't need to be negative — in fact, one of the most important keys to the program is learning to enjoy a full and active life.

Our ambitious subtitle is "conquering heart disease." The steps outlined in this book will help you dramatically reduce your risk of heart disease, even though it can't be completely eliminated. However, we believe that if you've done everything within your power to prevent heart disease or live with it as effectively as possible, then you have indeed "conquered" it!

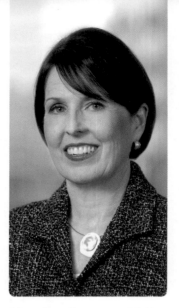

Martha Grogan, M.D.
Medical Editor

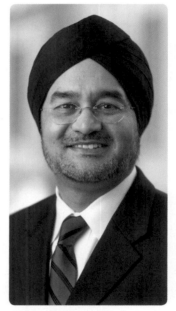

Charanjit S. Rihal, M.D.
Chair, Cardiovascular Diseases

How to use this book

This book can guide you to better heart health in 10 steps.

GET GOING!

Quick start your Mayo Clinic Healthy Heart Plan with Eat 5, Move 10, Sleep 8 — a catchphrase for three simple tasks on which you can take immediate action. Almost everyone can do it, and the sooner you begin, the better. The quick start prepares you for the full Mayo Clinic Healthy Heart Plan presented later in the book. Motivation is key — your full commitment to the program may be your most important predictor for success.

PART 1

10 STEPS TO HEART HEALTH

The Mayo Clinic Healthy Heart Plan identifies 10 factors that you can use to improve your heart health and reduce your risk of heart disease. Some factors call for lifestyle changes. Other factors involve a good working relationship with your doctor. Still other factors require you to have a greater awareness of how your heart works. If that seems like a lot to deal with, don't worry! There's nothing included here that you can't handle. Work at your own pace — this book guides and supports you every step of the way.

PART 3

IF YOU HAVE A PROBLEM

A heart condition likely won't stop you from using the Mayo Clinic Healthy Heart Plan. This section highlights six of the most common heart conditions and identifies ways that you can adapt the Healthy Heart Plan to meet specific needs of a condition.

SUPPORT YOUR PLAN

The opening parts of this book demonstrate the "how tos" of the Mayo Clinic Healthy Heart Plan. This part supplies some of the "whats" and "whys" — in-depth information that helps explain your actions. Chapters cover the basics of diagnostic testing, eating plans, exercise programs, finding a healthy weight, complementary and alternative medicine and mental health issues.

Your biggest risk

If you get nothing else out of this book, get this: Heart disease is the thing most likely to kill you — and there's a lot you can do about it.

Doing something good for your heart is the whole purpose of this book — to help you prevent heart disease or to help you live life to the fullest if you already have it. To that end, the Mayo Clinic Healthy Heart Plan is designed to guide you through a series of simple yet enjoyable changes to improve your heart health.

Being *enjoyable* is the key. You won't make the changes if you don't enjoy them. And you'll want to maintain these changes for a lifetime. So this book is big on enjoyment.

Another key to the program that may surprise you is the impact sleep has on your heart health. Combine quality sleep with eating healthfully and being physically active, and you have the major elements of the quick-start phase of this program — Eat 5, Move 10, Sleep 8. Doing all three elements well points you in the direction of a healthy, *enjoyable* life.

You'll get to the quick start in Chapter 1 soon enough, but first some preliminaries about why you should take heart health seriously.

Heart disease is the No. 1 killer in the United States. No one is immune. Here are some sobering statistics:

+ 80 million Americans have some form of heart disease — that's about 1 in 3 adults.

+ Every year, 2 million Americans have a heart attack or stroke.

+ Every day, 2,200 Americans die of heart disease — an average of 1 death every 39 seconds.

+ Heart disease kills more people each year than all forms of cancer combined.

+ Heart disease kills nearly five times as many women as does breast cancer.

+ About one third of Americans who die each year of heart disease are under the age of 75. It's not just an "old person's" disease.

+ Health care costs and lost economic productivity due to heart disease and stroke cost Americans an estimated $444 billion in 2010.

Heart disease does not discriminate. It can hit anyone, regardless of age, gender, race, social class or economic status. But there are some differences among the people who get the disease. Heart disease is generally more common among whites and blacks than it is among people of other races. African-American men and women are more likely to die from heart disease than are white men and women.

The good news is that most heart disease is preventable. Many risk factors for heart disease are factors you can change. If an emergency happens, prompt action can save your life. If you already have a heart condition, there's a lot you can do to make sure you live well despite your condition. The take-away message: You have far more control over your heart health than you may realize.

> " My wife saved my life by recognizing the early signs of a heart attack and getting me to the emergency room."

Jeff probably should have been aware of his risk of a heart attack. His father had diabetes and heart disease and died of a heart attack at age 62. An uncle died of a heart attack at 42. Jeff was a smoker and overweight — two major risk factors for heart disease. But still, his heart attack caught him by surprise.

Jeff had just finished eating lunch and wasn't feeling so hot. "I was getting restless — that's the best word for it," he says, recalling a December day nearly 30 years ago.

His wife, Millie, had just returned home from running errands when she noticed that Jeff seemed agitated. He would lie down, then get up and walk around, then lie down again. He kept clenching his left hand open and shut. "What's going on?" she asked him. He described pain down his left arm and told her he thought it was indigestion from a bowl of turkey soup he had eaten.

Millie also found a bottle of tooth pain reliever sitting out in the laundry room: "He had jaw pain, but he wasn't telling me." Millie worked as a nurse, so she knew what pain in the jaw and the left arm meant. She told Jeff, "I've warned you that if you're not careful, you're going to bite the big one. That's what's happening right now. You need to go to the hospital!"

Tests showed that Jeff had blocked coronary arteries and would require triple bypass surgery. Even after the procedure, Jeff had some rocky times when he and his doctors thought he might not make it. Fortunately, he has taken control of his condition. He is active and eating a healthier diet. "I look at the heart attack and everything I've been through as a positive," Jeff says. "I feel so much better. I probably never would have quit smoking. If I hadn't had the heart attack, I'm not sure I would've made it this far. I've got a prognosis for a good, lengthy life."

Warning signs of heart disease

We've all heard stories about someone like Jeff, who thought he had indigestion when it was actually a heart attack. Mistaking a heart attack for something else is common. In some cases, heart attacks and other heart problems do occur out of the blue, with no prior symptoms. But if you do experience any of the symptoms below, have them checked out.

✔ Chest pain or discomfort that you notice with physical activity or emotional stress, which goes away when you rest
✔ Unusual tiredness
✔ Shortness of breath during normal physical activities

Call for emergency help if you have:
✔ Unexpected chest pain or discomfort that doesn't go away after a few minutes or occurs when you're resting
✔ Discomfort in other areas of your upper body, such as your arms, shoulders, back, neck, jaw or stomach
✔ Shortness of breath that doesn't go away

Million Hearts

Heart disease is such a devastating — and preventable — disease that the U.S. Department of Health and Human Services has launched a major campaign to prevent 1 million heart attacks and strokes over 5 years. The program, a partnership of public and private organizations, launched in fall 2011. It will focus on empowering Americans to make healthy choices, on reducing the number of people who need medical treatment, and on improving care for those who do need treatment. For more on Million Hearts, go to: **millionhearts.hhs.gov**

✔ Severe weakness, lightheadedness, cold sweat or fainting
✔ Severe indigestion or heartburn that lasts more than a few minutes, feeling sick to your stomach, vomiting or abdominal discomfort

The symptoms may be subtle, especially in women. If you're not sure what's going on — but it feels different or troublesome — get yourself checked out. Don't delay! Delay can be deadly.

Renton Tech Coll Library

Common myths about heart disease

These misconceptions may keep you from making changes in your life now that may help you prevent heart problems later.

1 **'There's nothing I can do about it.'** Your dad may have died of a heart attack when he was 50, or you know several relatives who have heart problems. Does that mean you're also destined to get heart disease? No. Even if you have a strong family history of heart disease, there are effective ways to prevent it. This book contains many steps that can help you reduce that risk.

2 **'I don't have to worry. Heart disease doesn't run in my family.'** The flip side of believing you're fated to get heart disease is assuming you're protected because it's "not in my genes." Most of your risks stem from choices you make in your life, such as what you eat and how active you are.

3 **'Only old people get heart disease.'** It's true that your chance of getting heart disease increases as you get older. But many forms of heart disease actually take root in lifestyle habits formed during childhood — even in children, plaques can start to build up in arteries. Unfortunately, many young adults aren't concerned about heart disease and don't care that what

they're doing now can affect their lives later on. The best prevention program begins early in life.

4 **'I'll know if I have a heart problem because I'll have symptoms.'** Sometimes a heart attack is the first sign that there's any problem at all. Half the men and 64 percent of women who've had a heart attack showed no symptoms of heart disease before the attack. People with heart valve problems also may not experience symptoms.

5 **'Heart disease is more of a man's issue than a woman's issue.'** Though this myth has long been debunked, many women still fear breast cancer much more than they fear heart disease. But, in fact, heart disease is the leading cause of death and disability in women, just as it is in men. At the same time, women are less likely to make lifestyle changes to help prevent heart disease and they're generally reluctant to seek help with heart-related symptoms. Doctors add to the problem by not diagnosing heart problems as readily in women as in men.

6 **'I'll change my lifestyle if I get in trouble.'** If you have a heart attack, it might already be too late to make any meaningful changes — 15 percent of people don't survive a heart attack, and another 20 percent die in the year following the attack. Another thing to consider is your quality of life. Having a heart attack, living with cardiac symptoms such as chest pain and palpitations, or being treated for heart disease with medications, stents and bypass surgery is not reassuring for the future.

7 **'But I'm already living a healthy lifestyle.'** Maybe you really do lead a heart-healthy lifestyle. But, unfortunately, a lot of us think we're healthier than we really are. In a recent survey, 9 out of 10 college-age adults believed they were living a healthy lifestyle — when, in fact, they weren't. There's a frequent disconnect between what people know, say or believe about healthy behaviors and what they actually do. Just 3 percent of Americans regularly practice all four primary behaviors recommended for heart health not smoking, maintaining a healthy weight, eating a diet rich in veg-etables and fruits, and exercising regularly.

" You would think I would recognize the symptoms of a heart attack."

On what started out as a typical day, DeAnn, a medical secretary for the Cardiovascular Diseases Division, Mayo Clinic, began experiencing nausea, vomiting, sweating and arm discomfort — but no chest pain. The arm discomfort became so severe that at one point she thought, "I feel like I'm dying!" DeAnn was in her early 40s, healthy, active and had no history of cardiovascular problems — she couldn't believe the symptoms could be connected to her heart. DeAnn passed it off as food poisoning and resisted co-workers' advice to go to the emergency room. Eventually, she agreed to go. Tests showed she was having a heart attack due to an unusual cause — a condition known as spontaneous coronary artery dissection. Following stents to correct the problem, DeAnn has taken measures to resume her active life.

As the two patient stories illustrate, not recognizing the warning signs of a heart attack is an all too common occurrence. While Jeff didn't seem to take his risk of heart attack seriously, DeAnn had no known risk factors for heart disease. To get either of them to check out their symptoms took convincing from someone else.

Their stories illustrate the importance of knowing the signs and symptoms of a heart attack, no matter what your perceived risk.

Risk factors for heart disease

Your heart health starts with understanding your risks — taking an honest look at different factors that may increase the chance that you'll develop heart disease. A risk factor could be a medical condition, a behavior, a specific gene, or something in your environment — any of which, alone or in combination, could affect your heart health. Very often, if you already have heart disease, these risk factors increase the chance that your condition will worsen.

Of all the risk factors for heart disease, most are things you can do something about. Improving these factors is what the Mayo Clinic Healthy Heart Plan helps you do — take specific steps to change your risk profile and prevent future heart problems.

Using this book may also make you aware of being at risk of (or having) some of the heart conditions that can't be prevented. The bottom line is: The more you learn about heart disease, the more you can do something about it.

Here are some common risk factors for heart disease:

✔ High cholesterol levels
✔ High blood pressure
✔ Diabetes
✔ Obesity
✔ Smoking
✔ Lack of physical activity
✔ Age
✔ Personal or family history of heart disease

We'll provide more details about these risk factors — and how you can learn about which ones affect you — in later chapters of this book.

Why it matters

Why get all worked up about your risk factors for heart disease? Because getting a handle on your risk factors is a game-changer. During the last 30 years, deaths from heart disease have fallen by 50 percent — because more people were able to identify and treat their risk factors. The more you see heart disease as a real threat, the more motivated you'll be to do something to prevent it or to lessen its impact on your life.

The Mayo Clinic Healthy Heart Plan helps you start making the changes that will improve your heart health. You can start small. Even modest lifestyle changes can substantially reduce your risks.

It's never too late or too early to start. When you do, you'll also boost your overall health and longevity. And believe it or not, when you control your risk factors for heart disease, you reduce your risk factors for many other conditions, including dementia, cancer, diabetes, kidney disease, erectile dysfunction and blindness.

Are you ready to get started on a path to a healthier, longer life? Just turn the page.

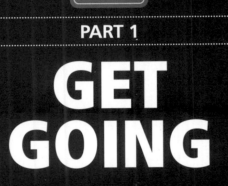

PART 1

GET GOING

Get started on the Mayo Clinic Healthy Heart Plan right now in an easy, two-week warm-up to the full program.

Eat 5

Boost your heart health by eating at least five servings of vegetables and fruits every day.

Move 10

Increase activity and exercise at least 10 minutes more than what you typically do every day.

Sleep 8

Get eight hours of sleep every night. Doing it for two weeks may get you hooked!

Many medical professionals may be involved in the treatment of heart conditions and support of healthy heart plans. This book often refers you to a doctor for care but would also like to acknowledge nurses, nurse practitioners, physician assistants, dietitians, physical therapists and others who play vital roles in keeping you healthy.

CHAPTER 1

GET READY TO START

It's so easy to take your heart for granted. Put your hand on your chest and feel the heartbeat — like a constant, steady companion. Maybe you know of someone who has had a heart attack or who has high blood pressure or another cardiovascular condition, and that's what has you worried about your own heart. You're ready to take steps to prevent the same thing from happening to you.

The introduction to this book just gave you reasons why you should be concerned about the health of your heart. Hopefully, you're ready to take action — and that's what the Mayo Clinic Healthy Heart Plan is all about.

There are many ordinary but very effective measures you can take to prevent heart disease. They're often part of routine activities you do every day. This is the basis of the quick-start approach: Simple actions that make an immediate, positive impact on your heart and provide long-term benefits to your health.

But before you begin the quick start, you need to figure out if you're ready. *Ready* means several things:

- ✔ Is it safe — physically — for you to start this plan?
- ✔ Are you motivated to make the changes in your life that allow you to be successful with this plan?
- ✔ Is right now the right time to start this plan?

This chapter helps you examine these three questions. Don't skip ahead until you've considered them.

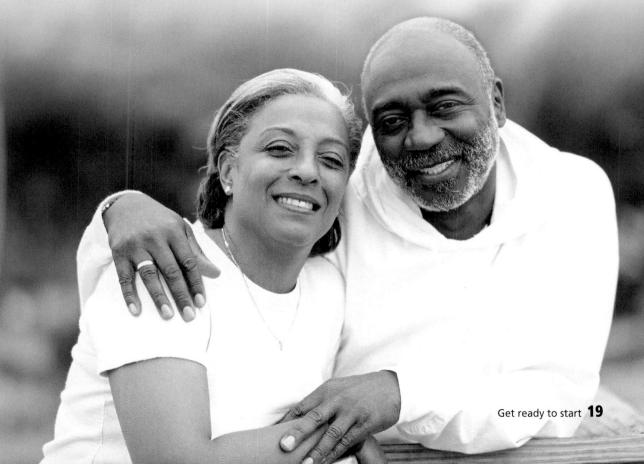

Do you need to see a doctor?

The quick start to the Mayo Clinic Healthy Heart Plan is appropriate for most people, but some should consult their doctor before beginning the plan. For example, if you're significantly overweight and have been inactive for several years, you and your doctor can choose activities that are safe and beneficial for you.

If any of the following statements apply to you, consult your doctor before proceeding with the quick start:

- You have a heart condition, and your doctor has recommended that you restrict your physical activity.
- You get breathless or experience chest discomfort or breathlessness at rest or with exertion.
- You have frequent dizzy spells or have had unexplained fainting episodes.
- You have severe muscle, ligament, tendon or other joint problems.
- You've been told to reduce your physical activity for any reason.
- You have uncontrolled high blood pressure.
- You're taking medications, such as insulin, that may require adjustment if you exercise.

Find your inner motivation

You'll learn the nuts and bolts of the Mayo Clinic Healthy Heart Plan in this book, but the most critical element of the plan is your motivation to improve your heart health. What's driving you to take action?

Why is motivation important? It's the internal force that gets you started in the first place. (Or rather, if you're unmotivated, you probably won't start the plan at all!)

The Mayo Clinic Healthy Heart Plan is going to involve some work and dedication. You're going to face obstacles, and your motivation will keep you going. Motivation carries you through periods of frustration, anxiety and boredom — all of which you'll experience at some point. It also helps you focus on the long-term goals of the plan.

The key to motivation is that it has to be personal. The reasons for taking action should be your reasons and not someone else's. The best motivation comes from within you, and without that internal drive, any goal — particularly a long-term goal such as heart health — will be difficult to achieve.

How do you discover your inner motivation? Start by asking yourself this question: "Why do I want to improve my heart health?"

Perhaps personal history plays a role, for example, a parent or sibling has had a heart attack. It could be that you're concerned about symptoms, such as fatigue or mild chest pain. Maybe you're interested in keeping a high quality of life for as long as you can. These are all strong motivators.

Maybe the facts and figures of heart disease have scared you. Fear is a great motivator. The point is: There are no wrong reasons for improving your heart health, as long as they are your reasons.

Write down all your motivators. With each entry, write down the specific reasons why they matter. Then find ways to keep these motivators in front of you, whether on Post-it notes or calendars or in email reminders. Be creative. Just as you came up with your own motivators, develop your own system of reminders for why you're improving your heart health. Doing so improves your chances of success.

Follow these steps for starting the Mayo Clinic Healthy Heart Plan:

+ Find your inner motivation. See the tips on this page for help.

+ Take the assessment *Are you ready to start?* on pages 22-23. Address any issues that may be challenges to your success.

+ Pick a start date. Before that date, familiarize yourself with the quick start and how to achieve the Eat 5, Move 10, Sleep 8 goals described in Chapter 2. Make preparations. For example, have vegetables and fruits on hand, and plan strategies for getting more physical activity and sleep.

+ On your start date, jump in and begin the two weeks of Eat 5, Move 10, Sleep 8 in Chapter 2.

+ Use a notebook to track your progress on how well you achieve the quick start goals.

+ Don't expect to be perfect — but try. You likely won't be able to achieve each goal on each day during the two weeks, but the closer you come, the better the results.

+ Consider asking a friend, relative or co-worker to join you in starting the plan. You might even consider a friendly competition. Sharing your commitment with others will increase your chance of success.

Are you ready to start?

There can be good times to start the *Mayo Clinic Healthy Heart Plan*, and there can be bad times. You don't want to put off your start date any longer than necessary, but you don't want to set yourself up for failure by starting at a time when you're facing major obstacles in your life.

Answers to the following questions can help you determine if now is a good time to start. If it's not, try to address those factors that seem to be interfering with your plans. After you've addressed those factors, set a start date to begin. Don't use these issues as a reason to continually put off improving your heart health — learn to deal with them.

1 **How motivated are you to make lifestyle changes right now to improve heart health?**
  a. Highly motivated
  b. Moderately motivated
  c. Somewhat motivated
  d. Slightly motivated or not at all

Knowing you need to make changes and feeling up to the challenge are two different things. To be able to cast aside established behaviors that affect eating, exercise, weight, or tobacco and alcohol use, you need to be motivated.

2 **Considering the amount of stress in your life right now, to what extent can you focus on diet, exercise, sleep and other lifestyle changes that improve heart health?**
  a. Can focus easily
  b. Can focus relatively well
  c. Can focus somewhat or not at all
  d. Uncertain

Having difficulty dealing with stress can make it hard to take on new challenges or be successful in making behavior changes.

3 Some heart-healthy goals, such as lowering blood pressure or cholesterol numbers, are a gradual, long-term process. How realistic are your expectations about how fast you want to achieve them?

a. Very realistic
b. Moderately realistic
c. Somewhat realistic
d. Somewhat or very unrealistic

Change may seem to move at an agonizingly slow pace, but if improving your heart health is a long-term goal, the speed at which it occurs won't matter.

4 Do you believe heart health is a lifelong commitment?

a. Yes, very much so
b. Yes, but I am more concerned about right now
c. I have never been able to stick to long-term goals

The most effective heart-health changes are permanent ones. Sure, you'll occasionally slip back to old habits and behaviors, but when that happens, you'll learn strategies that help you get back on course.

How did I do?

If most of your responses are a and b, you're probably ready to start the *Mayo Clinic Healthy Heart Plan*. If some of your responses are c and d, you may want to hold off on your start date and take action to prepare yourself for the program. For example, if you're unsure of your motivation, you may want to re-examine your reasons for wanting to improve heart health and explore new strategies to help you find your inner motivation. Or if you're experiencing a lot of stress, you may want to get that under control before starting the program. Your doctor may be able to help you address some of these issues to increase your readiness.

CHAPTER 2

EAT 5, MOVE 10, SLEEP 8

The preliminaries are over. Let's get started on the path to a healthier you. Welcome to Eat 5, Move 10, Sleep 8 — your two-week quick start to the Mayo Clinic Healthy Heart Plan. What you'll learn during quick start is heart healthy, for sure, but the quick-start approach will also help you enjoy life, another critical heart-healthy factor.

A quick start is just what it sounds like — it means you take immediate action. And Eat 5, Move 10, Sleep 8 are the goals upon which you take action. (More on those numbers later in the chapter.) The quick start lasts for only two weeks.

Sure, there's much more about heart health and disease prevention that you'll discover later — and this book guides you every step of the way — but the quick-start goals are important steps that you're taking right now.

During these two weeks, you'll learn that the process of making your heart healthier and stronger doesn't have to be complicated. Simple, everyday actions can help prevent heart disease. The key is turning them into habits.

Remember this is not a competition. Work at your own pace. Build your confidence and strengthen your commitment. You can prepare for the full Mayo Clinic Healthy Heart Plan by reading ahead in the book during the quick-start phase. And congratulate yourself that you're taking these initial steps. This effort can lead to a healthier, happier you.

Track your progress

Use a journal to track your progress during the quick start. This can be a simple notebook page marked off in columns and rows. For each day, put a check mark under each goal, if you've achieved it, or leave it blank if you didn't. At the end of two weeks, you'll analyze your results. For more on your scorecard, see page 30.

Don't necessarily expect to see progress for certain risk factors, such as a drop in your cholesterol. Those measurements typically take longer to change. But that's OK. The purpose of Eat 5, Move 10, Sleep 8 is to move you into a pattern of healthy living. Focus on consistently following the recommendations of the quick start. If you can do this, good results will follow.

So let's get started!

Step 1: Take a baseline quiz

Answering these three questions will give you a starting point for Eat 5, Move 10, Sleep 8. Your responses don't have to be exact — an estimate will do.

1. **How many servings of vegetables and fruits do you eat every day?**
   Give your answer from one to 10 servings.

   If your answer was five servings or more, you're in good shape for the quick start — and the higher the number of servings, the better. If your answer was four servings or fewer, you'll need to increase the number of servings.

2. **How many minutes each week do you take part in moderately intense physical activity?**
   Give your answer as follows: 0 = none, 1 = less than 30 minutes, 2 = 30-69 minutes, 3 = 70-109 minutes, 4 = 110-149 minutes, and 5 = 150 minutes or more.

   The more you're active, the better it is for your heart health. If your answer was 4 or 5, it means you're already pretty active. An answer of 2 or 3 means you could benefit from being

A word about serving sizes

Don't confuse servings with portions. A serving is a specific amount of food measured in cups or ounces. A portion is the amount of food you put on your plate. (There can be several servings in one portion.)

Use visual cues to estimate serving sizes. Think of a single vegetable serving as being about the size of a baseball. A single fruit serving is about the size of a tennis ball. That's all you need to know right now. For more on serving sizes, see page 45.

more active. An answer of 0 or 1 means you're not very active at all.

3. **How many nights out of the week do you get adequate sleep?**
   Give your answer from zero to seven days.

   This can be a subjective question — what feels like adequate sleep to one person is not enough to the next person. "Adequate" means you awaken easily in the morning feeling refreshed, and you remain alert during the day. Ideally, you want this on all, or at least most, days of the week. If your response is four days or fewer, getting more sleep should become a priority.

Step 2: Work on your goals

You're ready for the next stage of the quick start: Eat 5, Move 10, Sleep 8. It's true that everyone eats, moves and sleeps on most days. The quick start attaches specific numbers to these activities — and the numbers stand for daily goals you should reach:

- ✔ Eat 5 servings of vegetables and fruits.
- ✔ Move 10 minutes more.
- ✔ Sleep about 8 hours at night.

Don't worry right now about the whys and wherefores. You'll learn more about that later. For right now, just do them!

Follow these goals for two weeks. Use results from your baseline quiz to point out your strengths and weaknesses at the beginning. Even as you pursue your goals, read ahead in the book to prepare yourself for the full Mayo Clinic Healthy Heart Plan. Look to make these goals permanent habits.

A word about exercise intensity

Moderately intense means activity that causes you to perspire lightly and breathe a little more heavily. Examples include brisk walking, casual bicycling, water aerobics, ballroom dancing and general gardening. Exercise at more vigorous intensity includes jogging, fast bicycling, swimming laps, aerobic dancing and heavy gardening.

Don't forget to keep a simple log or checklist that indicates how well you're meeting your goals. Here are tips that may help you achieve them.

Eat 5 servings of vegetables and fruits

You may already know that vegetables and fruits are good for you — but how good are you at including them in your diet? It's not so hard with some attention and a little planning.

Start by eating breakfast and including at least one serving of fruit (or a vegetable, if you prefer). Eat a slice of melon or half a grapefruit, or add berries or banana slices to cereal or yogurt. The point is don't wait until dinner to fit in all of your servings of vegetables and fruits at once.

Never pass up a chance to add extra vegetables or fruit to a food you normally eat. This can be as simple as adding lettuce and tomato to your sandwich, or tossing a few frozen, cut-up vegetables into a soup you're warming up. Having vegetables and fruits available for between-meal snacks, for desserts or after you exercise helps cut back on other high-calorie options.

The good news is that there's no need to stop at five servings — that's a minimum number. In fact, the amount of vegetables and fruits you can eat in a day is unlimited. These foods are really that good for you! Go ahead and pick from a wide selection of types, colors, textures and flavors — the more variety, the better.

Move 10 minutes more

Add at least 10 minutes of moderately intense physical activity to what you already do every day. Official recommendations are for you to be active about 30 minutes a day on most days of the week. But the bottom line is, many people don't even come close to that amount.

If that sounds like you, then at least move for 10 minutes every day. That may not seem like much but studies show that doing 60 to 90 minutes of moderate physical activity a week may reduce your risk of heart disease by 30 to 50 percent! That's an incredible benefit from your effort.

Be honest with yourself — even on the busiest days, you should be able to fit a short activity break into your schedule. Once you get started, you may find yourself going longer than planned.

Walking is great because it's simple, safe, inexpensive, and you can do it almost anywhere. Yardwork, bike riding and dancing also count. Fit 10 minutes into your work routine, such as having "walk and talks" instead of sit-down meetings. Walk when you make phone calls, and exercise while you watch TV.

If you're already exercising regularly, focus the extra minutes on adding new kinds of activity to your program or doing more vigorous exercise.

Find new ways to move more. Be creative. Pursue activities that you enjoy. Once you get going, you'll realize that being more active is a little easier than you thought it would be.

Sleep about 8 hours at night

Sleep is something that many people claim they need more of but never have time for. It keeps getting squeezed out by a lifestyle of 24/7 communication and quest for success.

The quick start asks you to get eight hours of sleep every night. There's no denying that a good night's sleep restores energy and improves your disposition. Lack of sleep can make you prone to forgetfulness and fatigue. What you may not know is that quality sleep is good for your heart.

Quality sleep may require changing your bedtime routine. It may force you to turn off your cellphone and computer in the evening. You may have to learn how to relax. These are small changes that make a big difference.

Let's be clear, there's no magic number for how much sleep is optimal. Scientists have studied the question for years and recognize that sleep needs differ. A rare number of people can get along on little sleep, but studies show that most adults need between seven and nine hours every night.

Treat Sleep 8 as a general guideline. Depending on your circumstances, you may require a little more or a little less than eight hours. You'll learn about finding your "slumber number" later in the book, but for now, try to stay within the seven to nine hour range.

You might feel that there's no way you can find time to sleep that much. But convince yourself to make the effort for the next two weeks. Once you've tried it, you may find you actually like it!

Step 3: Check your scorecard

After two weeks, you can analyze your scorecard. The results may give you a better idea of what's most effective for you in establishing new habits or breaking old ones. Remember that what works for someone else might not work for you.

To analyze your quick-start results, review the log or journal that you kept as a guide. Follow these steps:

 Add up the total number of days you achieved each goal.

- ✔ Which goals were strengths for you?
- ✔ List reasons why you did well on those goals.
- ✔ Which goals did you not follow so well?
- ✔ List reasons why these goals were more challenging.
- ✔ Think of strategies for doing better with the challenging goals. Use resources elsewhere in this book for help. Come up with at least one strategy you can use right away. Write down all your ideas.

 Add up the total number of goals you achieved each day.

- ✔ On which days of the week did you do better?
- ✔ List reasons why you did better on those days.
- ✔ On which days did you not achieve your goals as well?
- ✔ List reasons why those days were more challenging. Try to identify patterns. Are there days of the week that pose special challenges?
- ✔ Think of strategies for doing better. Use resources in this book for help. Come up with at least one strategy you can use right away.

New beginning

You can hope that the results in your journal show one check mark for each goal for each day. But being perfect is unlikely, and perhaps unreasonable. At this point, you're aiming for consistency rather than perfection — achieving most of your goals on most days.

Don't become discouraged if you didn't hit every goal on every day. Just enjoy the success you've had and learn from your experience. Find ways to see how you can do even better.

The most important thing right now is that you've started the Mayo Clinic Healthy Heart Plan. You're taking the first steps of a lifelong journey toward better heart health. And that journey continues as soon as you turn the page to the next part of this book.

It bears repeating that the quick start is only the beginning. You've just put on walking shoes and headed out the door, but there's still a long and rewarding road ahead. There are many more things for you to learn about and do to improve your heart health. This book will provide you with the tools you need. For right now, celebrate what you've accomplished. Every little bit will, in the end, improve your heart health and reduce your risk of heart disease.

One more thing: The quick start lasted for two weeks, but don't let it end there. Don't plan on eating a few more vegetables for a couple of weeks, and then revert back to your old ways. Try to make a firm break from old habits while establishing new ones.

The Mayo Clinic Healthy Heart Plan is a lifelong plan. And if you care for your heart, there's no going back!

PART 2

10 STEPS TO HEART HEALTH

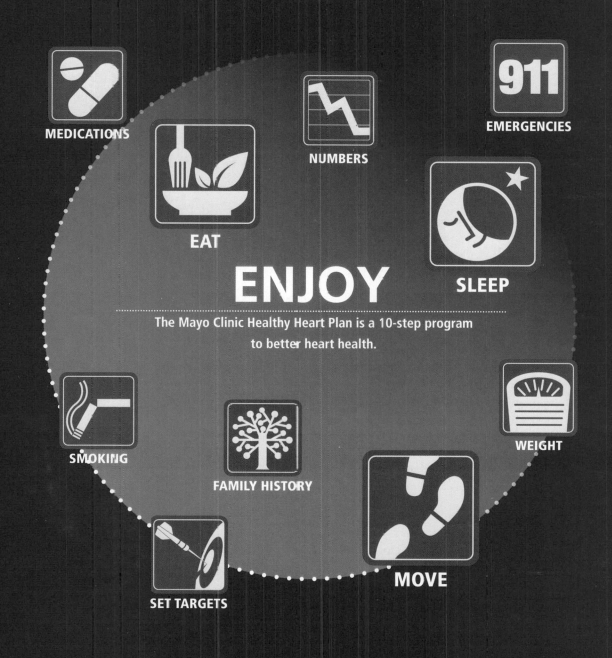

MEDICATIONS

EAT

NUMBERS

911
EMERGENCIES

SLEEP

ENJOY

The Mayo Clinic Healthy Heart Plan is a 10-step program to better heart health.

SMOKING

FAMILY HISTORY

WEIGHT

SET TARGETS

MOVE

Making the Mayo Clinic Healthy Heart Plan work for you

The Mayo Clinic Healthy Heart Plan is a step-by-step program that puts you on a path to better heart health. The 10 steps that make up the "heart" of the plan are shown on page 35.

Here's how you join the plan:

+ Each step of the healthy heart plan is treated in a separate chapter. (Tobacco use and weight are exceptions, because they're included in a single chapter.) Work on one chapter for one week — which means it will take 10 weeks to get through the plan completely. If you think one week per chapter is moving too fast or slow, adjust the pace to something that suits you better.

+ You're given three goals to work on every time you start a new chapter. You'll find these simple goals listed with this symbol:

+ Read each chapter carefully for important information and practical tips that will help you improve your heart health.

+ Try to accomplish the three goals as you work through the chapter. You can include other goals based on suggestions and ideas from what you've read. By the time you finish a chapter, you will have learned new tools that can improve your hearth health. It's OK if you haven't reached some goals by the time you're ready to move to the next step. Keep moving forward as you continue working on all your goals.

Each chapter provides you with an important piece of the plan. Once you've worked through all the chapters, you will have built a solid foundation for your healthy heart plan.

The important point is to "own" your plan. Make sure it fits your specific health condition, your priorities, your needs and your preferences. The right-hand columns on page 35 show what you can do.

At the end of 10 weeks, you'll be ready to chart your course for a heart-healthy future. Using the tools and knowledge you gained, you can continue to build your program and incorporate new strategies as you're ready.

Do the Mayo Clinic Healthy Heart Plan "by the book" or customized to suit your needs.
You can do the steps in the order provided by this book (example 1), moving through the chapters week by week. But let's say (example 2), you don't smoke, you have a healthy weight, and you've already taken a CPR class — so you can skip over chapters 6 and 11.

In addition, lack of physical activity is your biggest concern. If that's the case, start the program with Chapter 4, the activity chapter. In example 3, you don't smoke and you're not taking any medications. In addition, you're more comfortable with two weeks per chapter rather than one week. That's fine. Work at your own pace.

Eat healthy
Chapter 3

Be active
Chapter 4

Sleep well
Chapter 5

Deal with tobacco
Chapter 6

Deal with weight

Know your numbers
Chapter 7

Know your history
Chapter 8

Set your targets
Chapter 9

Take your medications
Chapter 10

Plan for emergencies
Chapter 11

Enjoy life
Chapter 12

Example 1

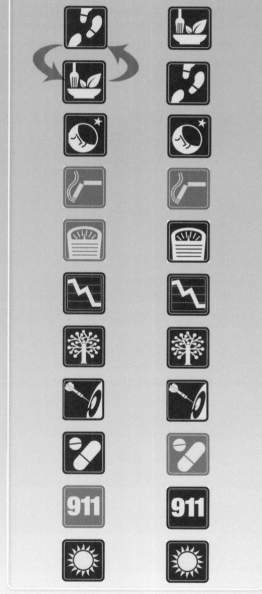

Example 2   Example 3

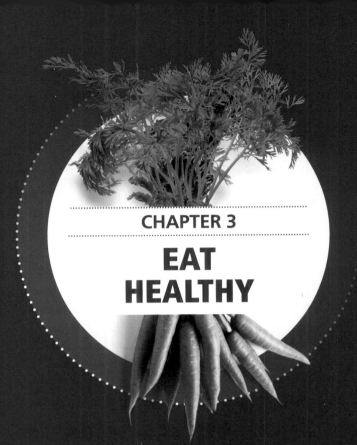

CHAPTER 3

EAT HEALTHY

Everyone can choose what to eat and how to eat. This chapter helps you know which choices may be the most meaningful for your heart health and your health overall.

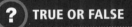 **TRUE OR FALSE**

Some types of dietary fat may lower your cholesterol.
- True
- False

True. The use of monounsaturated fats, such as canola, peanut, and olive oil are "good fats," and can lower your cholesterol.

Changing your diet can be a challenge. It's not that you can never eat a burger and fries again. Rather, your focus shifts to choosing healthier foods most of the time — a lunchtime salad, chicken or fish instead of red meat, an apple instead of a cookie for snack.

Some of the most important actions you take to improve heart health involve your diet and eating habits. What you eat raises or lowers blood pressure, blood cholesterol, and blood sugar, and it governs weight control. It can also reduce your risk of heart disease.

For example, take the goal from Chapter 2 of eating more vegetables and fruits. People who regularly eat five or more servings of vegetables and fruits each day cut their chances of heart attack and stroke.

It's time now to examine all aspects of your diet: What you eat, where you eat, how much you eat and how you prepare the food. You might find your way by trial and error or by taking two steps forward and one backward. But good eating habits will develop in the same way that some of your "bad" ones may have — you'll learn them.

I can DO this!

I'll build each step of my Healthy Heart Plan week by week with these simple goals:

+ Eat breakfast every morning, choosing whole grains, low-fat dairy, fruits and nuts and avoiding sugary cereals and baked goods.

+ Try one new heart-healthy recipe, and continue adding more recipes each week throughout the program.

+ Eat at least two meatless dinners each week.

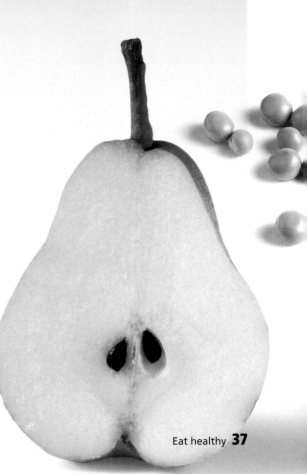

Eat healthy **37**

5 keys to a healthy diet and healthy heart

Use these key points to build a healthier diet. For more information on eating healthier, see Chapter 22.

① Boost your vegetables and fruits. Your mother was right when she insisted that you eat your broccoli. Vegetables and fruits are the foundation of a healthy diet. They're loaded with vitamins, minerals, fiber and antioxidants that may reduce your health risks. Vegetables and fruits are also low in fat and cholesterol.

Most people don't eat enough vegetables and fruits — in part because these foods seem less convenient, less affordable and not as easy to prepare as many fast foods and processed items. A common complaint is that vegetables taste bland. But you don't have to enjoy every kind of vegetable and fruit — just find the ones you like and eat those.

Buy vegetables and fruits that require little preparation, such as baby carrots, cherry tomatoes, broccoli, cauliflower, grapes, bananas and apples. Frozen varieties also come in handy as a quick addition to meals. Keep a bowl of fruit handy for easy snacking. Because of processing, fruit juice and dried fruits, such as raisins and prunes, can be a concentrated source of calories — eat them sparingly.

Use the following tips to add more vegetables and fruits to your diet:

+ Order or prepare main courses that feature plant foods — and use meat, dairy and other items to supplement the meal. Challenge yourself to have two or three meatless dinners every week.

+ While you're eating, work on your vegetable portions at the beginning of the meal, rather than reserving them for the end after you finish other foods and your stomach is beginning to feel full.

+ Add extra vegetables and fruits to foods you commonly eat. Throw a handful of vegetables into soup. Place fresh tomato, pepper and onion slices in a sandwich. Add fresh fruit to breakfast cereal, or stir the fruit in with yogurt or cottage cheese. Top small servings of dessert and pancakes with fruit.

+ Add a salad or vegetable soup to your lunch and dinner. Choose low-sodium canned soup or make your own. Use lots of fresh salsa when you have a craving for chips.

+ If you consider raw vegetables to be "rabbit food," lightly cook or roast them. Sprinkle them with herbs to boost the flavor. Or eat raw vegetables with a low-fat dip or natural peanut butter.

2 **Eat breakfast ... and eat it right.** Eating a healthy breakfast is one of the best ways to ensure that you have a varied, balanced and moderate diet. When you eat breakfast, you're more likely to get the vitamins, minerals and fiber you need for good health. Breakfast helps you control weight, reduce fat intake and lower cholesterol. You also may find that eating breakfast improves your concentration and productivity during the day.

To eat a good breakfast, even if you're not hungry, try these tips:

+ If you haven't been a breakfast eater in the past, change gradually. Have breakfast on two mornings of

Specialist focus:

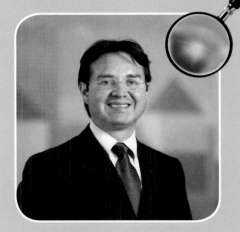

Francisco Lopez-Jimenez, M.D., is an expert in preventive cardiology at Mayo Clinic.

Nature gives us a lot of chances. For somebody who has many risk factors, it's amazing how just by becoming more active and eating better, many of the problems can get under control. Even if your body has been exposed to bad things for 30 or 40 years, six months of doing the right thing can lead to positive changes.

the week, and then aim for three mornings. Your eventual goal is to eat breakfast every day.

+ If time is an issue in the morning, do some preparation the evening before. Place a box of cereal, a bowl and a spoon on the table. Or have ready a breakfast shake that comes in a can or that you mix yourself.

+ Keep food on hand that you can carry with you to eat in the car, on the train or bus, or at work. Convenient on-the-go foods include apples, bananas, whole-grain bagels and low-fat yogurt in single-serving containers.

+ Choose breakfast carefully. Many breakfast cereals contain added sugar that you don't need. Avoid pastries, muffins and doughnuts, which typically are high in saturated fat and sugar.

+ If you don't like traditional breakfast foods, fix a breakfast sandwich.

3 **Go for the grains.** Grains, especially whole grains, are an essential part of a healthy diet. All types of grains are good sources of complex carbohydrates and key vitamins and minerals. Grains are also naturally low in fat. Better yet, they've been linked to a lower risk of heart disease.

When choosing grain products, look for the word *whole* on the packaging. Whole grains still contain the bran and germ, which are sources of fiber, vitamins and minerals. The refining process for flour strips out the bran and germ. And just because the word *wheat* appears on the packaging doesn't mean it's a whole grain.

Whole grains include whole-wheat bread, pasta and crackers, brown rice, wild rice, oatmeal, barley, bulgur, buckwheat, kasha, and popcorn.

Here are tips for including ample good grains in your daily diet.

+ Enjoy breakfasts that include whole-grain cereals, such as bran flakes, shredded wheat or oatmeal. Substitute whole-wheat toast or whole-grain bagels for plain bagels. Substitute low-fat bran muffins for sugary, white-flour pastries.

+ Make sandwiches using whole-grain breads or rolls. Swap out white-flour tortillas with whole-wheat versions.

+ Replace white rice with kasha, brown rice, wild rice or bulgur.

+ Feature wild rice or barley in soups, stews, casseroles and salads.

+ Substitute whole grains, such as cooked brown rice or whole-grain bread crumbs, to recipes for some ground meat or poultry.

+ Use rolled oats or crushed bran cereal in recipes instead of dry bread crumbs.

4 **Focus on fats.** Of all the changes that can make your diet heart healthy, reducing the amount of saturated fat and trans fat — think solid fats such as butter, margarine and shortening — in the food you eat may have the greatest impact. These fats raise your cholesterol levels and increase your risk of coronary artery disease, heart attack and stroke.

You shouldn't try to eliminate all fat from your diet — you need some for good health. But certain types of fat are better than others. Choose mono-unsaturated fats, such as olive, peanut and canola oils, or polyunsaturated fats, found in nuts and seeds. Just remember that all fats, good and bad, are high in calories.

A word on salt

Most people eat too much salt (sodium chloride) — almost twice as much as they need each day. Reducing your salt intake helps lower blood pressure and your risk of cardiovascular disease.

The table salt you shake on a baked potato or scrambled eggs is only a small amount of the salt in your diet. Most dietary sodium comes from processed foods you eat. The additives that help preserve food and enhance taste also are loaded with sodium.

Challenge yourself to eat more fresh foods and fewer processed foods. You may find that after gradually decreasing salt use, your taste buds will adjust and you'll prefer less salt.

When shopping, look for low-sodium or reduced-sodium options. In addition, limit your use of condiments that are typically loaded with sodium — such as salad dressings, sauces, dips and ketchup.

Foods from animal sources — meat, poultry, eggs, butter, cheese and whole milk — are major sources of cholesterol. The cholesterol in eggs is found in the yolks, not the whites.

To reduce unhealthy fats in your diet:

+ Limit the solid fats you add to food when cooking. Replace butter or margarine with olive, peanut or canola oils. Use nonstick cookware or vegetable oil cooking sprays. Saute vegetables in a small amount of water, broth or wine.

+ Top your baked potato with salsa or low-fat yogurt in place of butter or margarine, and use low-sugar fruit spread on your toast.

+ Check the labels of packaged foods. Some snacks — even those labeled "reduced fat" — may have trans fat.

+ Choose low-fat versions of milk, yogurt and other dairy products.

+ Cheese is a common source of saturated fat. Choose low-fat or reduced-fat versions, such as mozzarella and Parmesan, and eat in moderation.

5 **Be lean with protein.** Good sources of protein include lean meat, poultry and low-fat dairy products. But legumes — beans, peas and lentils — are good sources of protein and can be substituted for meat. They contain little fat and no cholesterol and are high in fiber.

If you really want to boost your heart health, eat more fish. The omega-3 fatty acids found in many types of fish, including salmon, mackerel, herring and trout, appear to reduce the risk of dying of heart disease. The American Heart Association recommends eating fish at least twice a week.

Many varieties of nuts, such as walnuts, almonds, hazelnuts and pecans, contain omega-3 fatty acids and can help lower cholesterol. But nuts are also high in calories — so a small handful is plenty.

Use these tips for including low-fat protein into your diet:

+ Incorporate meat substitutes into some of your favorite recipes, such as using vegetarian refried beans in burritos and tacos, or tofu in stir-fry dishes.

+ Trim visible fat from meat before cooking. Broil, roast, grill or bake the meat on a rack to allow remaining fat to drip away.

+ If you don't like the taste of fish by itself, include it as part of a larger dish, such as in soup or salad. Or choose a mild-tasting fish, such as tilapia, for making fish tacos.

+ Avoid eating fried fish. Instead, try brushing a fillet with a little olive oil and lemon or lime zest, or with mustard, and then grilling, baking or broiling it to perfection.

+ Poach fish or skinless poultry in broth, vegetable juice, flavored vinegar or dry wine. You can also cook fish in foil packets that seal in the flavors and juices.

+ Sprinkle a handful of chopped nuts into your dishes. Roasting them beforehand brings out a nice flavor and texture. Nuts also make good snacks, but they're high in calories.

Variety, balance and moderation

Base your daily food choices on three principles that are easy to remember and easy to follow: variety, balance and moderation. Including a wide variety of foods in your diet is the best way to get all the nutrients your body needs. A balanced diet means you're selecting adequate amounts of different kinds of foods — not too little and not too much of any one kind.

+ Eating in moderation means you're in control of portion size and not overeating. Even if it's healthy food, eating too much still creates too many calories.

+ "Variety" can mean eating from different food groups — vegetables, fruits, grains, meat and dairy — as well as eating different foods within each group. Your body needs many kinds of nutrients, and you can't get all of them from just a few sources.

+ Challenge your taste buds by trying foods you've never eaten before — perhaps it's papaya, tomatillo, chard or jicama. Set a goal of sampling at least one new food each week.

+ Don't get too hung up on exact daily serving goals. If you focus on the entire week, the fluctuations and missteps of your daily food choices will even themselves out.

+ Eat when you're hungry and not because you're feeling tired, lonely, angry or frustrated. Eating for reasons other than hunger often leads to overeating.

+ To control overeating, serve smaller portions and take slightly less than what you think you'll eat. Using a smaller plate or bowl makes less food seem like more.

+ Slow down between helpings — converse with your dinner partner, drink water or eat a piece of fruit. It takes about 10 minutes for your stomach to tell your brain that it's full. If you wait for the signal, you're less likely to overeat.

+ It's what you do 90 percent of the time that matters, not the occasional times you slip up or forget to do something. If you can stick with a healthy-eating pattern most of the week, give yourself an occasional treat.

Plates and serving sizes

The U.S. Department of Agriculture (USDA) released MyPlate to remind Americans to eat healthfully. Recommendations include filling half your plate with vegetables and fruit, using grain products that are primarily whole grains, switching to fat-free or low-fat dairy, and choosing foods with low-sodium content. For more about MyPlate, visit the USDA website at www.choosemyplate.gov.

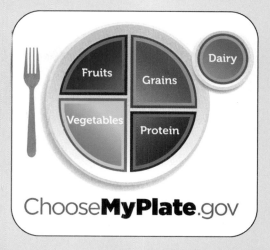

A food serving is an exact measurement and the size varies, based on the number of calories in a specific food. But you don't have to memorize or measure to get the serving sizes right. Use easy visual cues to estimate serving sizes on your own. For more on serving sizes, visit Mayo Clinic's website at www.mayoclinic.com.

1 vegetable serving =	1 baseball
1 fruit serving =	1 tennis ball
1 carbohydrate serving =	1 hockey puck
1 protein/dairy serving =	1 deck of cards or less
1 fat serving =	1 to 2 dice

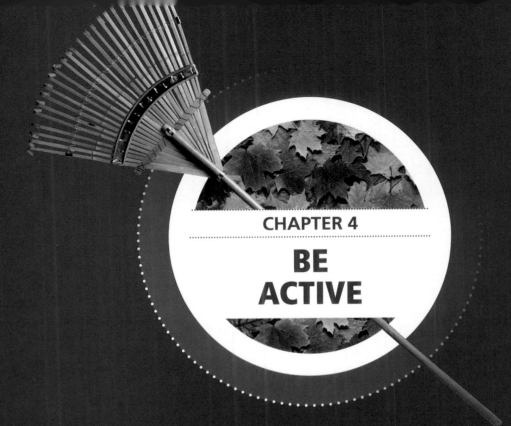

CHAPTER 4

BE ACTIVE

Of all the steps you can take for heart health, moving your body is one of the simplest and most important ones. You can start by literally taking a step.

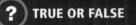 **TRUE OR FALSE**

Sitting for most of the day may be as bad as smoking for your heart.
- True
- False

True. Recent studies have shown that sitting for most of the day increases the risk of heart disease to a degree similar to that of smoking.

Being active can help you in many ways — improving sleep, weight control, concentration and mood. Regular exercise can help you control blood pressure and cholesterol and may reduce your risk of conditions such as heart disease, stroke, diabetes, osteoporosis, depression, Alzheimer's disease and erectile dysfunction.

The benefits of exercise apply to everyone — no matter what your age, weight, gender, race, health and fitness level. And the more active you can be, the more it can help you.

Many people incorrectly think that the only activity that will benefit their heart is a vigorous workout at the gym. But it turns out that you can dramatically reduce your risk of heart disease in much less time than you may have thought possible.

Even if you can't meet the recommended guideline of about 30 minutes a day, any exercise you do can help improve heart health and reduce your risk of disease. And once you get started, you may find that you want to do more — because it just feels good.

I can DO this!

I'll build each step of my Healthy Heart Plan week by week with these simple goals:

+ Find ways to turn 10 minutes (or more) each day of normal sedentary time into active time, for example, "walk and talk" meetings, short breaks to lift hand weights, and stationary bike rides while watching TV.

+ Participate in a new activity or exercise class that I've always considered interesting and fun.

+ Schedule regular exercise time throughout my week, including what, when, where and for how long I'll do it.

5 keys to physical activity and heart health

Use these tips to help you get more active. For more on physical activity and exercise, see Chapter 23.

 Stand up for heart health. Researchers have found that a sedentary lifestyle — spending a lot of time seated at a desk, in a car, or in front of a television or computer monitor — increases your risk of death from heart disease.

More alarming is the fact that this increased risk seems to be independent of how much exercise you actually do. Some studies have shown that among regular exercisers, those who spent the most time sitting when not exercising had a higher death rate than those who sat less.

Other studies have shown that the biggest drop in heart disease risk is achieved when someone goes from a sedentary lifestyle to being active for as little as one hour a week. You can do this just by "stealing time" during the course of a normal day. See "Get on your feet" on the next page for a number of easy options.

2 Start with 10. If you haven't been physically active for a while, don't expect to start exercising 45 minutes a day seven days a week. Begin with 10 minutes or so of moderate physical activity, such as a brisk walk — something that gets your heart pumping and makes your breathing faster but still allows you to carry on a conversation.

As you become more fit, spend more time and work a little harder on being active. You can increase the duration all at once or schedule short periods of activity throughout the day. Your eventual goal might be to be active for 30 minutes on most days of the week. Mix it up — work harder on some days and lighter on others.

+ Break up activity into small sessions, if you need to. Three 10-minute sessions offer similar benefits to one 30-minute session.

+ Remember that even low levels of activity are beneficial. Walk a dog, rake leaves, play a game of tag with your children or grandchildren — these activities don't take long but can make a big dent in your sedentary time.

Get on your feet

One very simple and effective way to give your heart a healthy boost is to reduce your sitting time. Here are just a few suggestions for fighting sedentary time in your daily routine.

At home

+ Get off the couch and walk around the house during TV commercial breaks. Or better yet, walk in place or use a treadmill or exercise bike while your program is on, or do household chores, such as folding clothes, washing dishes or ironing.
+ Stand to read your morning newspaper.
+ Wash your car by hand rather than using a drive-through car wash
+ Move around the house while talking on the phone.

At work

+ Stand and take a break from your computer every 30 minutes.
+ Take breaks from sitting time during long meetings.
+ Stand to greet a visitor to your workspace.
+ Use the stairs, even for just a few floors.
+ Stand during phone calls.

Source: National Health Foundation of Australia, 2011

+ Walk to your colleagues' desks instead of phoning or emailing.
+ Drink more water — going to the water cooler and restroom will help break up sitting time.
+ Use a height-adjustable desk so you can work while standing.
+ Have standing or walking meetings.
+ Eat your lunch away from your desk.

While traveling

+ Leave your car at home and take public transportation so you walk to and from stops or stations.
+ Walk or cycle at least part of the way to your destination.
+ Park your car farther away from your destination.
+ Plan regular breaks during long car trips.
+ Get on or off public transport one stop earlier than you could.

Specialist focus:

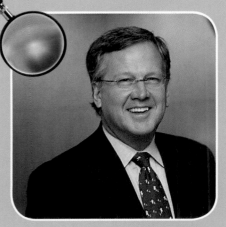

Stephen L. Kopecky, M.D., is a cardiovascular disease specialist at Mayo Clinic.

Try interval training a couple of days a week. During your workout, push yourself to a higher intensity for a brief period — only 30 seconds to start. It may be challenging, but it's quick! Back off and get your breath back, then do it again. As you get in better shape, your rest intervals will become shorter, and you'll be able to work out for a longer amount of time.

+ Warm up before any kind of exercise with easy walking. Allow time for recovery. Many people follow the "terrible toos" at first — too much, too hard, too fast, too soon — and soon give up. Plan time between activity sessions for rest.

+ Listen to your body. If you feel pain, shortness of breath, fluttering or rapid heartbeat, dizziness, or nausea, stop exercising. If symptoms persist or become worse, call your doctor. If you're not feeling well, take a day off — but get back to exercising as soon as you can.

3 **Add intervals.** Consider trying a technique that athletes often use to improve performance. Interval training involves alternating short periods of higher intensity activity with periods of lower intensity activity.

Interval training not only improves endurance — allowing you to exercise for longer periods — but also increases the number of calories you burn during exercise. It also appears to have a positive effect on helping to lower low-density lipoprotein ("bad") cholesterol and raise high-density lipoprotein ("good") cholesterol. An additional benefit of interval training is the change in routine, which adds variety and reduces boredom.

+ If walking is your exercise of choice, you can add interval training by starting out walking, then running or jogging for a few minutes, then switching back to walking. If you're less fit, you can alternate walking at a leisurely pace for a few minutes with walking fast. If you're a swimmer, try alternating a couple of fast laps with slower laps. The intensity and length of each interval are up to you and depend on how you feel and what your goals are.

+ If you have a chronic health condition or haven't been exercising regularly, consult your doctor before attempting interval training. Also keep the risk of overuse injury in mind. Try just one or two higher intensity intervals during each workout at first. If you think you're overdoing it, slow down.

+ As your stamina improves, challenge yourself to vary the pace. You may be surprised by the results.

An interval workout

Once you're able to exercise at a moderate intensity for 30 minutes, you can start to add interval training.

Start by alternating one to two minutes of moderate activity (such as brisk walking) with 30 seconds of hard activity (such as running). Include just one or two higher intensity intervals a session.

Here's an example of a 30-minute workout with intervals.

+ **Warm-up: 5 minutes**
+ **Moderate activity: 2 minutes**
+ **Hard activity: 30 seconds**
+ **Moderate activity: 2 minutes**
+ **Hard activity: 30 seconds**
+ **Moderate activity: 15 minutes**
+ **Cool-down: 5 minutes**

Over the next two to four weeks, two or three times a week, build up to three to five higher intensity intervals a session (on nonconsecutive days). Consider gradually increasing the length of the higher intensity intervals to 1 to 2 minutes each.

4 **Boost your strength.** Muscular fitness is another key component of an exercise program. Strength training at least twice a week can help you increase bone and muscle strength and reduce your risk of injury during activity. With regular strength training, you can reduce your body fat, increase your lean muscle mass and burn calories more efficiently.

You don't need to spend an hour or more each day lifting weights to benefit from strength training. Two to three sessions a week lasting just 20 to 30 minutes are sufficient for most people. You may enjoy noticeable improvements in your strength and stamina in just a few weeks.

+ Start slowly. Warm up with five to 10 minutes of stretching or gentle aerobic activity, such as a brisk walk. Then choose a weight or resistance level heavy enough to tire your muscles after about 12 repetitions.

+ Most fitness centers offer resistance machines and free weights. But you don't need to invest in a gym membership or expensive equipment to reap the benefits of strength training. Hand-held weights or homemade weights — such as plastic soft drink bottles filled with water or sand — may work just as well. Resistance bands are another inexpensive option. Your own body weight counts, too. Try pushups, abdominal crunches and leg squats.

+ To give your muscles time to recover, rest one full day between exercising each specific muscle group. When you can easily do more than 15 repetitions of a certain exercise, gradually increase the weight or resistance.

+ Remember to stop if you feel pain. Although mild muscle soreness is normal, sharp pain and sore or swollen joints are signs that you've overdone it.

5 **Pick things you enjoy.** Chances are, just knowing that physical activity is vital for good health is not going to motivate you to exercise. Likely, there's a recurring theme that goes along with thoughts of exercise — "I don't feel like exercising right now. Maybe I'll do it later."

The trick is to find out what it takes to get you moving. What interests you? What's fun? Make sure your workouts include things you enjoy.

+ Some people like to exercise on their own while others like group activities. Choose a form of exercise that suits your preference. If you like the chance to spend time with friends and family, try a dance club, hiking group or golf league, or sign up for a softball, soccer or volleyball team.

+ Reward yourself for small accomplishments. If you love music, treat yourself to a new song download after every exercise session. Give yourself extra relaxation time on weekends if you're able to fit short exercise breaks into your work days.

+ Focus on how good you feel when you exercise. Maybe it stems from a sense of pride or accomplishment or a boost in mood.

+ Enjoy the outdoors. If you love fresh air and nature, go outside and be active. Check out different parks for walking or biking. Try kayaking or rowing, or swim at the beach.

A new view

Some of the suggestions included in this chapter for being more active may be different from those you've heard over the years. Yes, it's great to be as physically active as possible, so if you're working out regularly, please don't stop! But let's face it — most of us don't come close to the recommended guidelines. Our lifestyles are so hectic that there never seems to be enough hours in the day. That's why simple strategies are provided here to weave activity into your daily routine.

Even if you're exercising consistently, make sure you're staying active throughout the entire day. Try adding interval training to increase your cardiovascular fitness and burn more fat. Make sure you do strength training to not only improve your physique, but also to prevent injuries and osteoporosis. This will allow you to enjoy an active lifestyle for years to come.

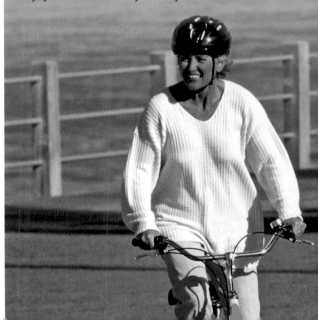

Make it a walk in the park!

Are you looking to ease into a regular walking program? This 12-week schedule from the National Heart, Lung, and Blood Institute can start you on the path to better health. Before starting this walking plan, talk with your doctor if you've been sedentary for a long time or you have serious health issues.

At first, walk only as far or as fast as you find comfortable. If you can walk for only a few minutes, let that be your starting point. For example, you might try several short daily sessions and slowly build up from there. Gradually work your way up to 30 to 60 minutes of walking on most days of the week. Over time, aim for at least 150 total minutes of moderate aerobic activity, or 75 minutes of vigorous aerobic activity, a week. Be sure to wear comfortable footwear with proper arch support and a firm heel. Also dress in loosefitting, comfortable clothing and in layers if you need to adjust to changing temperatures.

12-week walking schedule

Week	Warm-up (Slower walking)	Brisk walking	Cool-down (Slower walking)
1	5 minutes	5 minutes	5 minutes
2	5 minutes	7 minutes	5 minutes
3	5 minutes	9 minutes	5 minutes
4	5 minutes	11 minutes	5 minutes
5	5 minutes	13 minutes	5 minutes
6	5 minutes	15 minutes	5 minutes
7	5 minutes	18 minutes	5 minutes
8	5 minutes	20 minutes	5 minutes
9	5 minutes	23 minutes	5 minutes
10	5 minutes	26 minutes	5 minutes
11	5 minutes	28 minutes	5 minutes
12	5 minutes	30 minutes	5 minutes

Source: U.S. Department of Health and Human Services, 2006

Find a walking route

Many people like to have a planned route in mind when they go for a walk. That way, they can gauge how far they travel or how much energy they burn, while also feeling assured that the paths are safe and they won't get lost. You may prefer a loop (circular) path or an out-and-back path where you return along the same route on which you started. If you're not in shape, start with a 15-minute route, but try to work your way up to 30 minutes. Here are other guidelines to follow.

+ Plan a route that's close by and accessible. If possible, try to avoid long drives in order to exercise. Being able to step out your door to start your walk is both convenient and motivating. Use stores, downtown areas or public spaces as destinations.

+ Make personal safety your top priority. Try to walk in the daytime or in well-lighted areas. Carry a cellphone or whistle with you. Make note of locations along your route that may be useful, such as public restrooms, benches for rest, places to get out of the sun or rain, and stores that sell water.

+ Choose a route that's varied. Make it interesting, but don't involve too many stops, turns and busy intersections. You'll benefit most from a sustained, steady stride. Note where there are uneven sidewalks, inclines, loose gravel or dirt paths. Hills can add intensity to your walk, but include them at the beginning, while you're still fresh, rather than at the end of the walk.

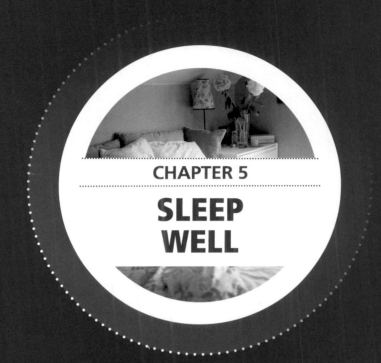

CHAPTER 5

SLEEP WELL

You spend about one-third of your life sleeping for a reason: It helps maintain good physical and mental health, reduces stress and re-energizes your body. But for many people, a good night's sleep is elusive.

? **TRUE OR FALSE**

Getting adequate sleep can help you lose weight.
- True
- False

True. Sleep deprivation promotes weight gain by stimulating appetite and depriving the body of quality sleep that may help you break down fat.

Are you constantly reaching for the snooze button on your alarm clock? Do you struggle to get out of bed in the morning? You're not alone. Our society pushes a busy lifestyle at the expense of sleep. In a recent poll, about two-thirds of Americans report feeling that their sleep needs are not being met. Unfortunately, sleep deprivation comes with a steep price for your health.

According to the Centers for Disease Control and Prevention (CDC), sleep deprivation has become a national public health epidemic. Chronic sleep deprivation impairs your attentiveness, coordination and reaction time. It also increases your risks of obesity, high blood pressure, heart attack, diabetes and depression. And sleepiness is the all-too-common cause of accidents and fatalities in the workplace and on the highways.

To get adequate sleep, something else has to give. Plan on spending less time working, watching TV or playing on the computer, and enjoy the blissful relaxation of a good night's sleep.

I can DO this!

I'll build each step of my Healthy Heart Plan week by week with these simple goals:

+ Set a bedtime and stick to it for the entire week, including the weekend. If I can't sleep as long as I want, I'll go to bed earlier.

+ Find relaxing things to do in the evening — light reading, listening to music, taking a bath — and make them part of my bedtime routine.

+ Turn off all of my electronic devices one hour before bedtime every night.

5 keys to sleep and heart health

Use these basic goals to improve your sleep and heart health.

1 **Aim for consistent quality sleep every night.** Even if you feel you get along just fine on little sleep, your biological need for it hasn't changed. It's a fact that most adults need seven to nine hours of sleep each night if they want to feel refreshed and stay in good health.

The amount of sleep you need is largely determined by heredity, and it varies throughout your life. Teenagers are programmed to sleep longer and stay up later, while older adults often develop just the opposite pattern. For most of your adult life, your sleep requirements are fairly constant and not something you can control. Less than 3 percent of adults function well on less than six hours of sleep.

Quality of sleep is just as important as the quantity of sleep. You can be in bed for eight hours and still feel drowsy the next day if your sleep is frequently interrupted during the night. When you sleep well, you wake up feeling refreshed, alert and able to carry out daily activities without being tired or dozing off.

To help you get enough quality sleep every night:

Learn your slumber number

Your slumber number is the number of hours you sleep at night that allows you to awaken in the morning without an alarm clock and feel refreshed. It also indicates the amount of sleep you should be getting regularly. Ideally, you should determine your slumber number when you're free of responsibilities, such as on vacation — but that's not always practical. Here's a method you can try: Determine what time you need to get up in the morning and go to bed seven or eight hours earlier. Try to wake up spontaneously without an alarm clock. Keep going to bed 15 to 30 minutes earlier until you can wake up without the alarm clock.

+ **Know your sleep patterns.**
  Keeping a diary for about 10 days
  helps you understand your sleep
  habits. Note when you go to bed,
  wake up, get out of bed, take naps
  and exercise. Also track your
  alcohol and caffeine consumption.

+ **Follow a sleep schedule.** Try to go
  to bed at about the same time every
  night and try to get up at about the
  same time every morning.

+ **Keep the same schedule on
  weekends.** It's best if your biological clock follows a consistent
  schedule. You can't sleep enough
  on Saturdays to repay "sleep debt"
  anyway. And changing your schedule on the weekend makes it harder
  to get back on track.

+ **Know your slumber number.**
  See page 58. You may not hit that
  number every night, but you have a
  goal to strive for.

2 **Get adequate sleep to help you
  lose weight.** Without enough
  sleep, you're more prone to weight
  gain. Lack of sleep stimulates your
  body to produce hormones that make

Problem sleepiness

You may not recognize the problem, but sleep is interfering in your
daily life if you:

+ Struggle to stay awake when
  you're inactive

+ Feel drowsy whenever you drive

+ Have problems with concentration and attentiveness

+ Have difficulty controlling emo-
  tions and you often feel
  irritable

+ Have slowed respons-
  es and memory
  problems

+ Crave sleep and
  feel fatigued
  most days

you feel hungry, and your body produces less of the substances that break
down fat. Because you're tired, you're
also less active. This is a sure recipe
for weight trouble. Making sure you
get an adequate amount of sleep can
help correct many of these problems.

Specialist focus:

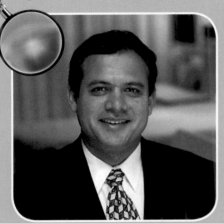

Virend Somers, M.D., Ph.D., is an expert on sleep and the cardiovascular system at Mayo Clinic.

You cannot sleep more than you need. If you're sleeping, it's because your body needs sleep. So don't cheat yourself. Sleep is a necessity, like food and water. It's not a luxury.

3 **Establish a consistent bedtime routine.** A relaxing routine just before bedtime helps you put aside the stress, excitement and hectic pace of daily life. Following this regular practice over time, you'll begin to associate restful behavior with sleep.

+ **Calm your mind.** Clear your mind of negative thoughts. Try to deal with worries earlier in the day. (Better yet: Worry less!) Read a relaxing book or magazine, take a warm bath, listen to music or reflect on good things that happened during the day.

+ **Create a quiet, dark, cool sleeping environment.** Block out or reduce outside noise. Get rid of all ambient light in the bedroom, including LED lights. Room temperature should be on the cool side.

+ **Turn off electronic devices.** This should be time reserved for yourself, not time for more stress and distractions.

+ **Don't eat a big meal just before bedtime.** A light snack is usually OK, but a full stomach or a heavy meal loaded with spices may cause discomfort during the night.

+ **Limit strenuous evening activity.** Regular exercise during the day promotes sleep, but strenuous evening workouts may have the opposite effect on some people, making it more difficult for them to fall asleep. Sexual intercourse is an exception to the rule, as intimacy helps promote sleep.

+ **Resist the urge to nap late in the day.** A midday nap is OK as long as it doesn't affect sleep at night, but avoid napping after 3 p.m. Generally, nap for only about 10 to 30 minutes.

4 **Be cautious about caffeine and alcohol.** Avoid coffee, tea and other sources of caffeine in the afternoon and evening. Caffeine is a stimulant that blocks sleep-inducing chemicals in the brain. Alcohol may actually help make you fall asleep, but it interferes with deep sleep and may cause you to wake up early. Avoid consuming alcohol less than three hours before bedtime.

5 **Make sure you don't have a sleep disorder.** As many as half of all people with heart failure may have some form of sleep apnea (see page 62). This sleep disorder is very common in people with high blood pressure, coronary artery disease and atrial fibrillation.

Sleep, obesity and heart disease

Sleep problems, obesity and heart disease often form a troublesome triangle, says Virend Somers, M.D., a Mayo Clinic cardiologist. "One condition leads to the other, which leads to the other, which leads to the other, with lots of interaction among them."

Obesity is a significant cause of sleep apnea, and many obese people have sleep apnea. Both conditions increase the risk of cardiovascular disease. All three sides of the triangle are linked to similar metabolic disorders such as diabetes, which in itself carries a high risk of heart disease.

On the plus side? Weight loss can improve all three conditions.

How do you know if you have a sleep disorder? Consult your doctor if:

▸ You snore very loudly or snore in a way that disrupts your sleep.
▸ You often feel sleepy during the day.
▸ You regularly wake up several times at night, including to pass urine.
▸ Your bed partner notices pauses in your breathing or sees you stop breathing during sleep.
▸ You often wake up with headaches, dry mouth or sore throat.
▸ You have high blood pressure or heart failure that's not improving with treatment.

People with heart disease should be especially careful about untreated sleep apnea, which increases the risk of death in people with coronary artery disease and heart failure.

If you're diagnosed with sleep apnea, a sleep specialist can outline treatment options. For mild cases, you may need to simply sleep on your side and not on your back. Weight loss is important for most people. Avoid sedatives, including alcohol, which make it easier for the airway to collapse during sleep. Many people use continuous positive

Sleep apnea

Obstructive sleep apnea is the most common form of sleep apnea. It occurs when soft tissue at the back of the throat sags while you're sleeping, blocking airflow through your windpipe for 10 seconds to a minute. You partially awaken, and the airflow starts again, usually with a loud gasp or snort. The cycle may repeat itself hundreds of times during the night.

Central sleep apnea — when the brain sends improper signals to the throat muscles — is much less common than obstructive sleep apnea. However, up to 40 percent of people with heart failure may have central sleep apnea.

airway pressure (CPAP), to manage sleep apnea. CPAP involves pressurized air pumped through a mask into your nose and throat to keep the airway open.

Some people with a mild form of sleep apnea or who cannot tolerate a CPAP mask may use an oral device similar to an orthodontic retainer to help keep their air passageway open.

Use a sleep diary

A sleep diary is a written record of how much and how well you sleep each night. The diary can help identify factors that disturb your sleep, be it from eating too much too late in the evening to being unable to let go of daily stress. You and your doctor may find the diary useful if you're dealing with conditions such as sleep deprivation, insomnia, snoring and sleep apnea.

Organize the diary however you like. Typically, you track sleep habits for at least one to two weeks. Each day you should record:

+ What time you went to bed at night
+ What time you woke up in the morning
+ Whether you woke up during the night

In addition, you should rate the quality of sleep on a scale of 1 (poor) to 5 (great). Much of the rating is based on how rested or tired you feel in the morning. Other information you may include:

+ Time of evening meal
+ Snacks before bedtime
+ Activities before bedtime
+ Stress level during the evening
+ Medication use
+ Alcohol or caffeine intake
+ Use of electronic devices

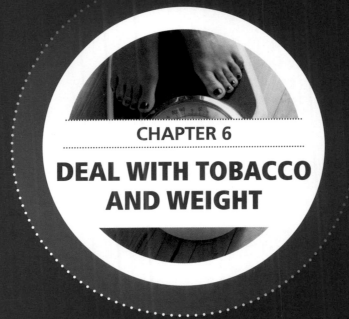

CHAPTER 6

DEAL WITH TOBACCO AND WEIGHT

These two factors are the elephants in the room. They're both big health risks, but no one wants to deal with them. They may be blocking your way to heart health. If you use tobacco or you're overweight, addressing either of these factors becomes a priority.

(?) TRUE OR FALSE

A healthy BMI (body mass index) is 32.
- True
- False

False. A BMI of more than 30 indicates obesity, a major risk factor of heart disease.

A question that may come to mind as you read this chapter: Why are two topics as significant as tobacco use and weight loss being paired together?

Primarily because the knowledge you need on how to quit tobacco or lose weight is so extensive that it's not possible to provide it in detail here. You can find a wide variety of practical information, tools and support for tackling either issue from many government agencies, professional organizations and medical institutions.

The primary goals of this chapter are to raise your awareness of the impact of tobacco and weight on your health, and to direct you to resources that can help you begin to address the problem.

Unlike other heart-healthy steps such as diet, exercise and sleep, quitting smoking and losing weight don't apply to the entire population — not everyone is a smoker and not everyone needs to lose weight. So, this chapter may not be as important to you as other chapters. On the other hand, if you do smoke cigarettes or struggle with your weight, this chapter has great significance.

I can DO this!

I'll build each step of my Healthy Heart Plan week by week with these simple goals:

+ Write down three reasons why I want to quit smoking or lose weight. Make my reasons personal — not what someone else wants for me.

+ Enlist three family members or friends who are willing to support me as I try to quit smoking or lose weight.

+ Pick a start date to quit tobacco or lose weight.

Tobacco and heart health

Cigarette smoking is the leading preventable cause of death and disease. Millions of Americans develop lethal or debilitating conditions, including heart disease, because they smoke or have smoked in the past. Smoking damages several organs and tissues, and can make chronic conditions such as asthma worse. In short, tobacco affects just about every aspect of your health.

Tobacco use has a powerful effect on your cardiovascular system. Smoking narrows your blood vessels, raises blood pressure and increases the risk of blood clots. Any tobacco use — including smokeless tobacco — increases your risk of heart attack and stroke. Even "social smoking," one or two cigarettes a day, increases the chance of heart disease. Being exposed to secondhand smoke increases your risk of heart disease by 25 percent or more.

Resources for quitting smoking

Toll-free tobacco quit lines are available in every state in the United States and many countries throughout the world. Call the national quit line at 800-784-8669 to find the best fit for you. These online resources can also help you:

American Cancer Society
www.cancer.org

American Heart Association
www.heart.org

American Lung Association
www.lungusa.org

Ex
www.becomeanex.org

Mayo Clinic Nicotine Dependence Center
www.mayoclinic.org/ndc-rst

National Cancer Institute
Free Help to Quit Smoking

www.cancer.gov

Nicotine Anonymous
www.nicotine-anonymous.org

QuitNet: Quit all together
www.quitnet.com

Smokefree.gov
www.smokefree.gov

The good news is, quitting tobacco brings immediate benefits. Within 20 minutes of smoking that last cigarette, your heart rate drops. Within a year, your risk of heart attack is cut in half. Within two to three years, your risk is the same as that of a nonsmoker.

How do you quit smoking?

You can start by picking a quit day. Choose a day within the next two weeks so you'll have time to get ready but not so much time that you lose motivation. Ask your doctor to help build a quit-smoking plan and provide you with the most appropriate medication. Seek support from family and friends.

Many people find a two-pronged approach to be the most effective way to quit tobacco use: Combine quit-smoking medications with support from a tobacco treatment specialist or behavior counselor. A treatment program sponsored by a hospital, health care plan or employer may also be beneficial.

Counseling helps you develop life skills to break the addiction cycle and stay away from tobacco over the long run. Quit-smoking products ease the withdrawal symptoms of nicotine.

Specialist focus:

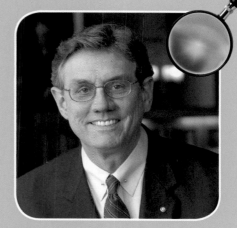

Richard D. Hurt, M.D., is an expert on tobacco cessation at Mayo Clinic.

Stopping smoking is a process that doesn't happen all at once. Start with manageable amounts of time, and work your way up to a whole day without smoking. Then take it one day at a time. Don't attempt it all on your own — there are many resources that can help you.

Medications include over-the-counter nicotine patches, gum and lozenges, as well as prescription nasal sprays, inhalers and pills. Medications help control nicotine cravings and reduce the pleasurable effects of smoking.

Weight and heart health

Over the last 30 years, obesity rates have skyrocketed across the world. More than two-thirds of American adults are now overweight or obese, as are almost one-third of children. The reasons for the epidemic are straightforward — people are eating more and being less active.

Being overweight or obese increases your risk of heart disease and conditions that lead to heart disease,

including high blood pressure, high cholesterol and triglyceride levels, diabetes, and sleep apnea. Obesity also puts you at risk of other chronic health conditions, including asthma and arthritis, as well as some cancers.

Losing weight reduces or reverses many of these risks. If you've been successful with the plan of Eat 5, Move 10, Sleep 8 in this book, you're on your way to a healthy weight. It

 Resources for losing weight

Some people prefer to lose weight on their own. Others benefit from the encouragement of a support group or formal program. No matter what your preference, there are resources available to help you. Look for options that teach you how to make positive changes in your life, encourage realistic goals, and link you to qualified professionals. *The Mayo Clinic Diet*, a book from Mayo Clinic weight-loss experts, can help you get started (www.store.mayoclinic.com). Also check these online resources:

Centers for Disease Control and Prevention
www.cdc.gov/healthyweight

Department of Agriculture
www.choosemyplate.gov

Dietary Guidelines for Americans
www.health.gov/dietaryguidelines

National Heart, Lung, and Blood Institute
www.nhlbi.nih.gov/health/public/heart

National Weight Control Registry
www.nwcr.ws

Physical Activity Guidelines for Americans
www.health.gov/paguidelines

We can!
www.nhlbi.nih.gov/health/public/heart/obesity/wecan

doesn't take much — losing just 5 to 10 percent of your current weight may lower your risk of heart disease.

What if I need to lose weight?

How do you know if weight is putting your health at risk? Check the body mass index (BMI) table on page 257. Generally, if your BMI number is 24.9 or less, your weight is probably fine. If your BMI number is 25 or more, you're likely overweight or obese and could benefit from weight loss. Consult your doctor about your BMI, weight goals and appropriate steps you can take to reach them.

Use the Mayo Clinic Healthy Weight Pyramid to build your weight program (see also chapters 22 and 24). The pyramid guides your food choices while also promoting physical activity.

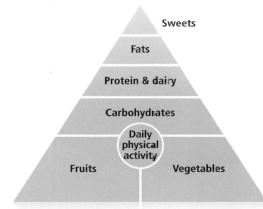

Specialist focus:

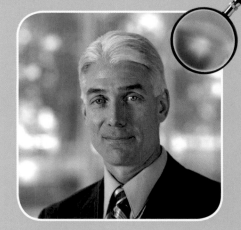

Donald D. Hensrud, M.D., is an expert on nutrition and preventive medicine at Mayo Clinic.

Much of your success with weight loss is in the planning. Don't focus too much on a long-term goal of losing 40 pounds — it won't happen without a plan. Trying to lose 40 pounds without a good weight loss plan is like trying to make a million dollars without a good financial plan. Instead, concentrate on losing one pound at a time. Many people also find that when they lose weight and are more active, they feel better.

8 strategies for getting started

Regardless of whether you plan to quit smoking or lose weight, there are certain strategies that can help you get started toward either goal. The keys to success are good preparation and having a plan to carry you through.

1. **Make sure you're ready.**

   Quitting smoking and losing weight can take time and effort. You want to make sure you're committed and focused before dealing with either. Starting too soon, before you're ready, can set you up for failure. Consider other stresses in your life, such as financial problems or relationship conflicts, and address them to a point where you feel they're under control. Only you can decide when you're ready.

2. **Find your personal motivation.**

   No one else can make you quit smoking or lose weight. You need to have your own reasons. Find out what gives you an ongoing, burning desire to change. Are you worried about the health consequences of smoking or obesity? Do you want to look and feel better or sleep more restfully? Maybe you need to set a good example for your family. Perhaps you want to breathe easier or save a little money or fit better in your clothes. Make a list of what's important to you and carry it with you to help stay motivated.

3. **Choose your approach.**

   There's no single "right way" to stop smoking or lose weight that everyone can use with success. If you've tried to do either in the past but failed, think about what worked or didn't work and what you'd be willing to try again. Consider all options and come up with a plan that you're comfortable with.

4. **Involve your doctor.**

   Your doctor or a member of his or her staff can review your overall health status, fitness level, medical conditions and medications to help you set realistic goals that make sense for you and that you can achieve. Ask about the need for additional counseling from specialists.

5. **Get support.**

   Get others to work on your side. Tell family, friends and co-workers of your plans to quit tobacco or lose weight. Although ultimately you're responsible for your own behavior, it helps to surround yourself with people who will encourage you, listen to your concerns, and share the priority you've placed on a healthier lifestyle. Your support network also offers accountability that helps you stick to your goals.

6. **Tackle one change at a time.**
If you're obese and you smoke, don't try to quit smoking and lose weight at the same time. That will overwhelm you. Consider focusing on quitting tobacco — with its almost instantaneous health benefits — as your top priority (while trying to not gain more weight).

7. **Manage your stress.**
Stress and anxiety can derail your efforts to quit smoking or lose weight. They undermine your commitment, sap your energy and distract you from meeting your goals. To keep stress under control, prioritize your tasks for the day, and consider which you can eliminate or delegate to someone else. Take a break when you need it and learn to relax.

8. **Pick a date.**
Choose a start day to quit smoking or lose weight. Account for circumstances in your life that may hamper your efforts, such as work deadlines, school exams, family obligations or vacations. Have a specific day in mind. Don't set the date too early or too far in the future — you may find it hard to follow through.

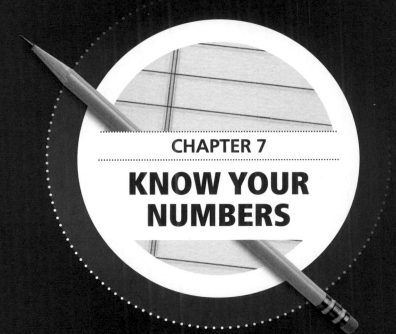

CHAPTER 7

KNOW YOUR NUMBERS

In preceding chapters, the focus of the Healthy Heart Plan has been on changing your lifestyle habits, such as diet, exercise and sleep. In this chapter, you're being asked to schedule a few simple medical tests. The results of these tests are referred to collectively as "your numbers."

(?) TRUE OR FALSE

If you do not have high blood pressure by age 55, your risk of developing it later in life is about 50 %.

- True
- False

Answer: False. The lifetime risk of developing high blood pressure for middle-aged adults in the U.S. is 90%. One third of those are unaware of their condition.

It just takes a phone call to your health care provider to schedule the tests you need for a heart checkup. You may ask, "If I'd like to check on my heart health, what tests would you recommend?" Your doctor will advise you.

The basic tests, including those for blood pressure and cholesterol, are common ones — they're often part of a general physical exam. But even if you've had some of this testing done in the past, it's still best to have recent test results. These numbers help establish a baseline of your current health and direct the next steps you take.

This chapter highlights the value of having a good working relationship with your doctor. The level of trust and honesty that develops will help both of you when interpreting test results.

Knowing your numbers can be especially important if you're a woman. Women are less likely to be treated for heart disease than are men — in part because heart disease may not be on many doctors' radar, and because diagnosing heart disease in women can sometimes be trickier than in men (see, for example, page 85).

I can DO this!

I'll build each step of my Healthy Heart Plan week by week with these simple goals:

+ Calculate my body mass index (BMI) and measure my waistline.

+ Write down my test results for blood pressure, cholesterol, triglycerides and blood sugar. If I haven't had these tests recently, I'll schedule a medical visit to do so.

+ Start a chart or table to track my numbers, including the next recommended follow-up visit.

5 numbers for better heart health

Numbers associated with the following tests can help identify your potential risk of heart disease: Blood pressure, cholesterol, triglycerides, body mass index, and blood sugar.

1 **Blood pressure.** Blood pressure measures the force of circulating blood that's pressing against your artery walls. The harder your heart pumps and the less flexible your artery walls become, the higher your blood pressure.

High blood pressure (hypertension) damages and scars the arteries. It's one of the major risk factors for heart disease. If not treated, high blood pressure can cause a heart attack, stroke or heart failure.

Nearly one-third of U.S. adults with high blood pressure don't even realize they have it. Most people show no signs or symptoms. African-Americans are at greater risk of high blood pressure than are whites.

The only way to know if you have high blood pressure is to be tested. Starting at age 18, have your blood pressure checked every two years. You may be screened earlier if you have additional risk factors. If you already have high blood pressure, your blood pressure will be checked more often.

The test. Blood pressure is generally measured with an inflatable arm cuff and a pressure-measuring gauge. A blood pressure reading, given in millimeters of mercury (mm Hg), has two numbers — sometimes stacked one on top of the other like a fraction:

+ The top number measures the pressure in your arteries when your heart beats (systolic pressure).

+ The bottom number measures the pressure in your arteries between heartbeats (diastolic pressure).

A doctor generally takes readings at two or more visits before giving a diagnosis of high blood pressure. That's because blood pressure varies from day to day. It can vary with exercise, sleep, stress and even posture changes.

2 **Cholesterol.** Your body needs cholesterol — a waxy substance found in the fats (lipids) carried in your bloodstream — to build healthy cells. But too much cholesterol causes fatty deposits to build up in your blood vessels. This can lead to narrowed or blocked arteries (atherosclerosis), a major cause of heart disease. Most people with high cholesterol feel fine and don't experience signs or symptoms. Being tested and knowing the test results is the best way to keep cholesterol levels within healthy limits.

The test. A complete cholesterol test, called a lipid panel or lipid profile, measures how much cholesterol and triglycerides you carry in your bloodstream.

Blood pressure categories

Top number (systolic) (numbers in millimeters of mercury)	Bottom number (diastolic)	Category
Under 120 &	Under 80	Normal
120-139 or	80-89	Prehypertension
140 & over	90 & over	Hypertension

If your systolic pressure is 115 mm Hg and your diastolic pressure is 78 mm Hg, your blood pressure is written as 115/78 and spoken as 115 over 78 — putting you in the normal blood pressure category (under 120/80). If the two numbers fall into different categories, the higher category is where you're placed. For example, if your test results are 125/78, you may be placed in the prehypertension category.

After age 50, the systolic number becomes more significant. Isolated systolic hypertension (ISH) — when the bottom number is normal but the top is high — is the most common type of high blood pressure among older adults, especially women. Prehypertension often leads to hypertension and puts you at risk of developing heart and blood vessel disease. Extremely high blood pressure — readings of 180/110 and over — can be life-threatening and requires emergency medical attention. (See page 108 for more on dangerously high blood pressure.)

> **" I'd been having chest pains.
> I thought it was heartburn..."**

Name: Ravuth

Event: At age 24, Ravuth visited the emergency room after experiencing shortness of breath and chest pain whenever he walked. Tests revealed extensive blockage of his coronary arteries. Ravuth had to have quadruple bypass surgery.

Outcome: Ravuth learned he has familial hyper-lipidemia (FH), an common inherited condition of extremely high cholesterol levels. His father died of a heart attack several years earlier. Ravuth's family didn't realize they had FH, a condition that should be suspected in people who have heart attacks early in life, before age 50 or 60. Children in families with FH should have their cholesterol checked starting as early as age 2. As for Ravuth, he's exercising without any problems now. His experience has helped him become healthier and more positive. "It can be a debilitating disease and hard to cope with sometimes, but I'm alive, I'm happy, and it's taught me not to stress out about the little stuff."

(We'll get to triglycerides later.) The simple blood test determines:

+ **Low-density lipoprotein (LDL) cholesterol.** This is sometimes called "bad" cholesterol. Too much of it in your blood causes athero-sclerosis. The deposits can rupture, leading to heart attack or stroke.

+ **High-density lipoprotein (HDL) cholesterol.** This is sometimes called "good" cholesterol because it helps carry away excess LDL choles-terol in your blood.

+ **Total cholesterol.** This is a sum of your blood's cholesterol content.

You may given a number for non-HDL cholesterol — which accounts for all forms of cholesterol minus your HDL cholesterol (there's more than just LDL and HDL cholesterol). This number may be a better indicator of heart risk than your LDL result alone.

All adults age 20 or older should have a full lipid profile taken once every five years. If you already have high cholesterol levels or a family history of early coronary artery disease, your doctor may ask for more frequent testing. New guidelines recommend checking cholesterol in all children between ages 9 to 11, and earlier in families with a strong history of heart disease.

Cholesterol is measured in milligrams of cholesterol per deciliter (mg/dL) of blood. The numbers categorize your risk level for heart disease, as shown in the chart below.

LDL cholesterol (in milligrams per deciliter)

Under 100	Desirable or optimal
100-129	Near optimal or above optimal
130-159	Borderline high
160-189	High
190 & over	Very high

HDL cholesterol

Under 40	Low
Over 60	Desirable

Total cholesterol

Under 200	Desirable
200-239	Borderline high
240 & over	High

These categories may not be in step with the cholesterol goals recommended by your doctor. For example, if you have heart disease, your doctor may ask that you aim for LDL cholesterol below 70 mg/dL.

③ Triglycerides. Triglycerides are another type of fat in your bloodstream. When you eat, your body coverts calories it doesn't immediately need into triglycerides. High triglyceride levels are common in people who are overweight or have diabetes, don't exercise regularly, eat too many sweets and carbohydrates or drink too much alcohol. Triglyceride levels above 200 are linked to an increased risk of death from cardiovascular disease.

The test. Triglycerides are measured in milligrams per deciliter of blood (mg/dL), and are normally included in a full cholesterol test. Triglyceride levels are generally higher during pregnancy.

Triglycerides (in milligrams per deciliter)

Under 150	Normal
150-199	Borderline high
200-499	High
500 & over	Very high

4 **Body mass index.** You may know that being overweight increases your risk of heart disease. But how do you know if you're overweight?

Weight is typically measured by a number known as your body mass index (BMI), which takes both your weight and height into account. Find out your BMI by using the chart on page 257. Your BMI number indicates whether you're at a healthy weight or you're overweight or obese.

BMI

18.5-24.9	Normal weight
25.0-29.9	Overweight
30.0-39.9	Obese
40 & over	Extremely obese

BMI isn't a perfect measure of healthy weight. Critics say it underestimates obesity, particularly among white and Hispanic women. It can also mistakenly label athletes with lots of lean muscle mass as obese. Talk to your doctor about your BMI number and whether you need to improve it.

Measure your middle. Another important weight-related number to know is your waist measurement. Fat around your middle is an independent risk factor for heart disease. If you have a large waistline, your risk of heart disease is high, even if your BMI is normal. Compared with fat in your legs or buttocks, belly fat has more dangerous health consequences.

A waist measurement of more than 35 inches (89 cm) for women or more than 40 inches (102 cm) for men is considered high risk. You can't just "spot reduce" your belly fat, so work on overall weight loss. As you lose weight, your waistline will shrink.

5 **Blood sugar.** Blood sugar (glucose) is your body's main fuel source. If dangerous levels of blood sugar build up in your bloodstream, you can develop diabetes. Because the signs and symptoms come on gradually, you might have high blood sugar without even knowing it. If you have diabetes, controlling your blood sugar level helps you feel your best and prevents further complications, including heart disease.

The test. The main test for diagnosing diabetes is a fasting plasma glucose test. It involves analyzing the level of blood sugar in a small sample of your blood after an overnight fast. The American Dietetic Association recommends that all adults age 45 and older be tested every three years. People with risk factors for diabetes should be tested earlier and more often.

If your test results are above normal, your doctor will repeat the test on a different day. If your blood sugar falls consistently in the range of 100 to 125 mg/dL, you're considered to be at high risk of developing diabetes. This condition is sometimes called prediabetes and is linked to a higher risk of heart disease.

Fasting blood glucose (in milligrams per deciliter)	**Category**
99 & under	Normal
100-125	Increased risk or prediabetes
126 & over	Diabetes

A blood sugar level that is consistently at 126 mg/dL or higher generally means you'll be diagnosed with diabetes. The disease can damage major arteries as well as small blood vessels, increasing your risk of heart attack, stroke and other disorders from impaired blood circulation.

Specialist focus:

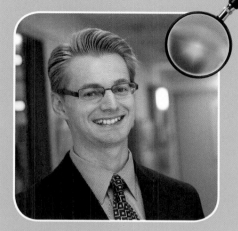

Regis Fernandes, M.D., is an expert in cardiovascular disease at Mayo Clinic.

A key to preventing heart disease is proactively seeking information to reduce your risk. It starts with a general physical examination. If individuals, health care providers and society worked together, most heart attacks could be prevented.

If you have diabetes, the glycated hemoglobin, or A1C, test can indicate how well you've been managing your blood sugar over the previous two to three months. You're doing well if the test shows that your average glucose level has been at 5.7 percent or lower.

Questions for your doctor

The test results described in this chapter can guide the decisions you make for improving your heart health. But the tests are not ends in themselves — don't get tested one time and then forget to be tested again. Testing should be repeated on regular occasions (see the table on page 81). Here are questions you may ask your doctor during medical visits:

- Are my blood pressure, cholesterol and blood sugar at healthy levels?
- How are my current blood pressure and cholesterol levels affecting me?
- Am I at risk of diabetes? Should I check my blood sugar at home?
- How often should I have blood pressure, cholesterol and blood sugar tested?
- What is a healthy weight for me?
- What changes can I make to improve my numbers?
- Do I need additional screening tests for heart disease?

Metabolic syndrome

A cluster of risk factors, known in combination as metabolic syndrome, greatly increase your risk of heart disease. You have metabolic syndrome if you have three or more of the following:

+ Waist circumference of more than 35 inches for women or more than 40 inches for men

+ Triglyceride level of 150 mg/dL or higher, or you're receiving treatment for high triglycerides

+ HDL cholesterol level of 40 mg/dL or less in men or 50 mg/dL or less in women, or you're receiving treatment for low HDL

+ Blood pressure higher than 130 mm Hg systolic or 85 mm Hg diastolic, or you're receiving treatment for high blood pressure

+ Fasting blood sugar of 100 mg/dL or higher, or you're receiving treatment for high blood sugar

If you have metabolic syndrome, work with your doctor to develop an aggressive plan to improve and maintain your numbers.

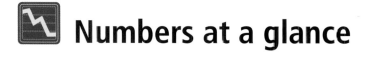

Numbers at a glance

Test or measurement	What the numbers mean	How often needed
Blood pressure	Under 120/80 mm Hg – Normal 120-139 80- 89 – Prehypertension 140/90 & over – Hypertension	Every 2 years, or more often if recommended
Cholesterol	**LDL** Under 100 mg/dL – Desirable or optimal 100-129 – Near optimal or above optimal 130-159 – Borderline high 160-189 – High 190 & over – Very high **HDL** Under 40 mg/dL – Low Over 60 – Desirable **Total** Under 200 mg/dL – Desirable 200-239 – Borderline high 240 & over – High	Every 5 years, or more often if recommended
Triglycerides	Under 150 mg/dL – Normal 150-199 – Borderline high 200-499 – High 500 & over – Very high	Every 5 years, or more often if recommended
BMI	18.5-24.9 – Normal weight 25.0-29.9 – Overweight 30.0-39.9 – Obese 40 & over – Extremely obese	Several times a year
Waist size	35 inches & over (women) – High risk 40 inches & over (men) – High risk 31 inches & over (Asian women) – High risk 35 inches & over (Asian men) – High risk	
Blood sugar (fasting plasma glucose)	99 mg/dL & under – Normal 100-125 – Increased risk or prediabetes 126 & over – Diabetes	Every 3 years starting at age 45, or earlier if recommended
Blood sugar (A1C)	5.7% & under – Normal 5.7-6.4% – Increased risk or prediabetes 6.5% & over – Diabetes	

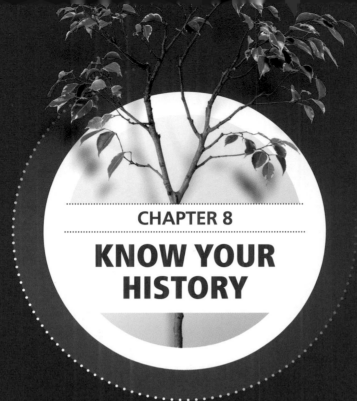

CHAPTER 8

KNOW YOUR HISTORY

To prevent problems in the future, you may need to look at the past. Find out what to look for in your own medical history — and that of your family — to better understand your risk of heart disease.

(?) TRUE OR FALSE

High cholesterol can be inherited.
● True
● False

True. High cholesterol can be inherited. The most common condition is called familial hyperlipidemia.

Did you know that a condition that has affected you or a family member in the past may be a strong predictor of your future health risks? For example, having a close relative who developed heart disease at a young age increases your chance of heart disease.

That may sound scary, but don't panic! Just because certain genes increase your risks doesn't mean you can't lessen those risks. There are things you can do to reduce your risks, including adopting a healthier lifestyle. It's important to check your medical history.

Personal history

Building your medical history starts at home, but consulting your doctor is very helpful. While some factors, like a heart attack, may be an obvious risk, other red flags, such as sleep apnea, anemia or kidney disease, might not show up on your radar.

Your doctor can also help you interpret how risk factors interact with each other. You might be aware that diabetes increases your risk of heart disease, but do you know the impact on your heart if you're also overweight?

I can DO this!

I'll build each step of my Healthy Heart Plan week by week with these simple goals:

+ Make a complete list of first-degree relatives (parents, siblings, children) and second-degree relatives (grandparents, uncles, aunts, nephews, nieces). If known, include birth dates and, if applicable, death dates.

+ Find out if a close relative had a heart attack at a young age (for men, under age 55 and for women, under age 65). Find out if any close relative experienced unexpected sudden death or cardiac arrest.

+ Get ready to start building a medical history by contacting relatives and asking for their help in answering the questions on pages 87-88.

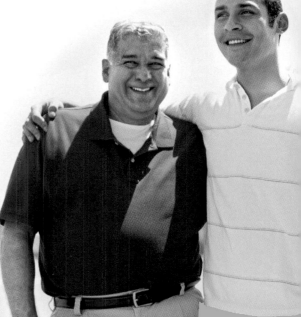

If you've regularly seen a health care provider over the years, your medical records will be useful. Regardless, be prepared to answer questions about illnesses, surgeries, health concerns and lifestyle. Prepare notes before the visit, including everything you know about your history — it doesn't have to be complete. A current list of the medications and supplements is important.

 ## Clues to your heart disease risk

A variety of diseases and conditions in your family or personal history may increase your risk of heart disease. Let your doctor know if you or a close relative has ever experienced:

+ Heart and blood vessel disease, including aortic aneurysm or dissection, cardiomyopathy, coronary artery disease, heart failure, heart valve disease, long QT syndrome, Marfan syndrome and peripheral artery disease

+ Heart attack (including angioplasty or stent placement), heart surgery or heart damage

+ Birth (congenital) heart defects, including bicuspid aortic valve

+ Stroke

+ High blood pressure

+ Diabetes

+ High or abnormal cholesterol levels

+ Elevated lipoprotein (a) levels

+ Depression

+ Alcoholism or other substance abuse

+ Miscarriage, stillbirth or pregnancy complications

+ Long-term kidney disease

+ Sudden death while in seemingly good health

Factors that increase your risk if they happen only to you:

+ Heart infections

+ Sleep apnea

+ Obesity

+ Metabolic syndrome

+ Rheumatic fever

+ Anemia

+ Thyroid problems

Women's unique risks

Women have specific issues to consider when reviewing their medical histories:

Pregnancy complications. A condition such as preeclampsia typically goes away after delivery, but you're left with a higher risk of high blood pressure and heart disease. Inform your doctor if you had gestational diabetes, preterm birth or an infant who was small for his or her gestational age.

Oral contraceptive use. Low-dose birth control pills generally don't increase heart disease risk in women under age 30. However, the risk for women smokers who take the pills is high, especially if they're older than 35.

Postmenopausal hormone therapy. Doctors once thought hormone therapy might help reduce the risk of heart disease in postmenopausal women. However, clinical trials indicated that estrogen not only doesn't reduce the risk, but also has other potentially harmful effects. Despite the results of these trials, many women continue using hormone therapy to reduce menopausal symptoms. Talk to your doctor before considering its use.

Autoimmune diseases. Rheumatoid arthritis and lupus are examples of autoimmune diseases, when the body's own immune system attacks healthy tissue. Autoimmune diseases occur more often in women than in men and significantly increase the risk of cardiovascular disease.

Other concerns. Women are more likely than are men to have diabetes. In fact, diabetes is a major risk factor for heart disease in women. Depression, which is more common in women, is another concern. The American Heart Association recommends screening women for depression as part of a regular cardiovascular evaluation.

Family history

Just as traits such as curly hair, brown eyes and musical ability may run in families, so does a tendency to get heart disease.

You inherit half of your genetic profile from each parent. In addition, your family typically shares a common home environment and lifestyle that can make a direct impact on your heart health.

Specialist focus:

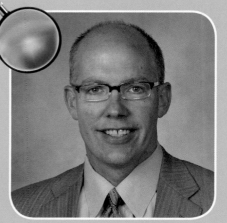

Michael J. Ackerman, M.D., Ph.D., is an expert on inherited and genetic heart rhythm disorders at Mayo Clinic.

Preventing sudden cardiac death in children relies on three strategies: Don't ignore abrupt fainting episodes, especially during exercise. Know your family history. Encourage your community to make easy access to external defibrillators a priority.

Researchers haven't untangled all of the different genetic and environmental factors involved, but they do know that your risk of heart disease increases if:

+ Your father or brother developed heart disease before age 55

+ Your mother or sister developed heart disease before age 65

Many people may think, "Well, if my dad died young of a heart attack, then heart disease is in my genes and I can't change that." Not so. The life you lead — your environment — plays just as big of a role as your genetic heritage in influencing your risk of heart disease. Nature and nurture work in concert — and the way you live your life can actually modify your genes.

At the other extreme, people can deny a family history of heart disease. "My dad may have died of a heart attack, but it's not happening to me!" These individuals may even ignore alarming symptoms, such as chest pain.

Acknowledging your family's medical history can help you identify patterns outside of your own personal experience. Similar to a genealogical tree, building a family medical history becomes a record of your extended family's health and reveals subtle relationships across the generations.

Your family history may not predict the future, but it will indicate factors that you need to be concerned about. You can acknowledge them and lessen their impact by changing unhealthy behaviors and staying on top of your numbers.

Getting the facts. To begin collecting a medical history, check to see if family members are willing to work together on the project. Always allow the option to answer questions privately by phone, mail or email. Either way, keep your questions short and to the point.

As you collect information, listen without judgment or comment. Not everyone feels comfortable disclosing personal information. Respect the right to confidentiality. Inform relatives that participation is optional and the information will be shared only with a medical professional.

For earlier generations, you may need to consult family trees, baby books, old letters, newspaper obituaries or records from places of worship. Birth certificates, marriage licenses and death certificates are usually available in county record offices.

If you're adopted, ask your adoptive parents if they received information about your biological parents. Adoption agencies also may keep family information on file. With an open adoption process, you may be able to consult your biological family directly.

Compile information about grandparents, parents, uncles, aunts, siblings, cousins, children, nieces, nephews and grandchildren. The first-degree relatives — parents, children and siblings — have the most direct impact on your heart risks. If possible, include at least two previous generations along with the current one in your history.

You can start your history by recording the sex and date of birth of each person you interview. Then ask them these questions:

- ✔ Do you have a chronic health condition, such as heart disease, high blood pressure or diabetes?
- ✔ Have you ever had serious illnesses, such as cancer or stroke?
- ✔ How old were you when you developed these conditions?
- ✔ Has your health been affected by factors such as diet, exercise,

weight, or the use of tobacco, alcohol or drugs?

✔ What medications do you take?

✔ Have you or your partner had any difficulties with pregnancy, such as miscarriages?

✔ What diseases did our deceased relatives have? How old were they when they died? What country did our ancestors come from?

Your personal and family histories don't need to be complete, but they do need to be as accurate as you can make them.

Sharing personal and family histories with your doctor provides valuable information about your risk of heart disease. In addition, your doctor will find the information helpful for recommending treatments or lifestyle changes that reduce your risk, scheduling ongoing screening tests, identifying other family members who may be at risk, and assessing your risk of passing conditions on to your children.

Making a family medical tree

Create a diagram or chart that clearly shows the relationships among various family members. If you don't have information about a disease or cause of death, don't guess at the answer — that may lead to a wrong interpretation. Don't worry if some details are missing.

Online tools are available that may help you. Go to the following organizations and type "family history" into the search function:

+ Department of Health and Human Services (*familyhistory.hhs.gov*)

+ American Medical Association (*www.ama-assn.org*)

+ National Society of Genetic Counselors (*www.nsgc.org*)

Give your doctor a copy of your record. Update the history every couple of years, and share the updates with your doctor.

"We're just like everyone else — we want to live life to its fullest."

On a spring morning, Michelle received a call at work from her son's school. Shannon, age 17, hadn't shown up that day. When Michelle's father checked on him, he found Shannon dead in his bedroom. The family's world turned upside down.

Shannon had seemed perfectly healthy. "We had annual physicals. We ate balanced meals. Autopsy reports showed no evidence of drugs and no apparent reason for cardiac arrest. No one could tell us what happened," said Michelle. The lack of an explanation puzzled her. "I had worked as an emergency medical technician and had been taught that you would know if a patient was sick enough to die." Several months later, Michelle discovered a valuable clue. While reviewing a copy of Shannon's sports physical, Michelle noticed Shannon had checked yes to questions regarding dizziness, chest pain and trouble breathing during and after exercise.

Those responses prompted Michelle to call her doctor, who ordered tests for her other son, Dustin. The abnormal results prompted mother and son to see a team of Mayo Clinic cardiologists. They discussed the family's health history, which included heart palpitations in Michelle's sister, as well as incidents of fainting in both Michelle and her mother. Genetic testing revealed that Michelle and Dustin both had long QT syndrome, a hereditary heart rhythm disorder that can cause fast, chaotic heartbeats and fainting, seizures or death. A molecular autopsy of Shannon's heart tissue confirmed the same genetic defect.

Michelle and Dustin received implantable cardioverter defibrillators (ICDs) to prevent the development of life-threatening heart rhythms. "We want to keep doing everything we can," says Michelle. "I want Dustin to be successful and just have fun, too. I don't want long QT to stop us."

CHAPTER 9

SET YOUR TARGETS

Your objective is to prevent heart disease, but how do you plan for such a long-term, complex goal? This chapter helps you set a course for reaching it.

(?) TRUE OR FALSE

The common risk factors for heart disease, such as smoking, high cholesterol, and high blood pressure also increase the risk of dementia and erectile dysfunction.

● True
● False

True. Smoking, high cholesterol and high blood pressure increase the risk of dementia, erectile dysfunction, breast cancer and some other cancers.

Test numbers and medical histories have helped you and your doctor assess the current state of — as well as potential risks to — your heart health. Now, your focus can be turned to the future and how to influence it for the better. You'll begin collaborating with your health care team to set targets — the long-term goals that help reduce your risk factors for heart disease.

To start, it might help to understand the difference between an "outcome" goal and a "performance" goal. An outcome goal is an end result, such as reaching an LDL cholesterol level below 100 mg/dL or losing 30 pounds. This type of goal is a big-picture or long-term goal that you may have to work on for a while.

A performance goal is a type of goal that helps you achieve the outcome, for example, "I will eat four daily servings of vegetables" or "I will walk 30 minutes every day" (either of which may help you lower cholesterol or lose weight). You typically need to identify several performance goals to meet an outcome goal. And for your healthy heart plan, you'll need to identify both outcome and performance goals.

I can DO this!

I'll build each step of my Healthy Heart Plan week by week with these simple goals:

+ Calculate my 10-year risk of heart disease by using a risk calculator such as the one on the National Cholesterol Education Program website. I'll discuss the results with my doctor.

+ Determine my top three outcome goals (targets), with my doctor's help.

+ Identify a series of performance goals that will help me achieve one outcome goal.

Specialist focus:

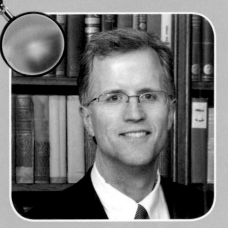

Randal J. Thomas, M.D., is an expert in preventive cardiology at Mayo Clinic.

There's a saying that heart disease is what nature gives you for breaking its rules. But you have a second chance. Healthy lifestyle habits can help you reduce a majority of your risks for heart attack.

Your targets should be based on your personal risk factors for heart disease. In collaboration with your doctor, determine what are the next steps you should take.

Your personal risk

In reviewing your personal risk factors, your doctor may use a risk-profile report to advise you on specific factors. The doctor may describe your overall risk level as being desirable (the level at which you want to be), moderate, high or very high.

Many people will have at least one risk factor for heart disease. The more factors you have, the more cause for concern. That's because one factor tends to reinforce the impact of other factors, multiplying your risk.

Fortunately, you can do something about many risk factors. For example, the chances of a 53-year-old male smoker with high blood pressure to have a heart attack over the next 10 years is about 20 percent. But if he stops smoking, his risk drops to 10 percent. If he takes high blood pressure medications, his risk drops to 5 percent.

The more you reduce risk, the bigger the payoff. If by age 50 you have your cholesterol and blood pressure under control, you don't smoke, and you don't have diabetes, your risk of heart disease over your lifetime is less than 5 percent.

What's your chance of a heart attack in the next 10 years?

Have you wondered what your chances are of having a heart attack or stroke? Tools called risk calculators help predict the likelihood. The result is expressed as a percentage, for example, a 20 percent chance, within a certain amount of time, such as 10 years.

In the United States, the most common risk calculators are based on the Framingham Heart Study that identifies factors contributing to cardiovascular disease. These tools generally require information about your age, sex, upper (systolic) blood pressure number, cholesterol level, and whether you smoke or have high blood pressure.

Try an online calculator from the National Cholesterol Education Program website (nhlbi.nih.gov/about/ncep) by entering "risk calculator" into the search function. The calculator is designed for adults age 20 and older who don't have heart disease, diabetes or familial hypercholesterolemia (FH).

All risk calculators have limitations. For example, they typically do not include family history or the presence of metabolic syndrome into the calculation. They may underestimate risk in women. Most calculators give your 10-year risk, not your lifetime risk, so you may be falsely reassured. Even if your risk score is low — say, 1 percent — you could be that 1 in 100 individuals who has the heart attack. Since the original Framingham study included only white adults, it may not apply as well to risk in nonwhite populations. Finally, most risk calculators give an estimate of your risk of heart attack or stroke, but not of other important heart conditions, such as atrial fibrillation or heart failure.

Researchers continue to study and learn more about risk factors, and new risk calculators are being developed to incorporate new findings. Your doctor may advise you if additional laboratory or imaging studies are needed to further assess your cardiovascular risk.

Major risk factors for heart disease

Diabetes. Having diabetes doubles the risk of heart disease in men and triples the risk in women.

Smoking. The more you smoke, the more likely you are to have a heart attack.

High blood pressure. This condition, especially if it's uncontrolled, can lead to plaque buildup and thickening or hardening of your arteries.

Unhealthy cholesterol levels. High levels of low-density lipoprotein (LDL) cholesterol or low levels of high-density lipoprotein (HDL) cholesterol increase your risk of heart disease. High levels of triglycerides also increase risk.

Family history of early heart disease. Your risk goes up if a close relative developed heart disease at an early age (before age 55 in men and 65 in women) — especially if he or she had no clear risk factors, such as tobacco use or high blood pressure.

Obesity. Being obese can lead to high blood pressure, high cholesterol and diabetes — all risk factors for heart disease. Carrying excess weight around your abdomen is especially bad for heart health.

Lack of physical activity. While regular physical activity helps protect you from heart disease, inactivity nearly doubles your risk. In fact, a sedentary lifestyle carries almost as much increased risk of a heart attack as does smoking.

Established heart disease. If you've had cardiovascular disease, including heart attack, stroke, abdominal aortic aneurysm, coronary artery disease, or chest pain, you're more likely to develop additional problems.

Other risk factors

Advancing age. Being older than age 60 is a risk factor for cardiovascular disease. Atherosclerosis already starts developing by age 20 in many individuals in Western societies and progresses over time.

Unhealthy diet. Eating too little of healthy foods, such as vegetables and fruits, and eating too much of unhealthy foods high in fats and sugar can raise your risk.

Sleep problems. Not getting enough sleep can lead to high blood pressure and obesity, both major risk factors for heart disease. Sleep apnea is linked to a higher risk of heart disease.

Stress. Stress can have an indirect and a direct effect on heart disease risk. When you're under stress, you may turn to overeating, heavy drinking or smoking to cope, all of which add to heart disease risk. In addition, chronic stress alone can have a direct damaging effect on the heart. Furthermore, a stressful or emotionally upsetting event is a common trigger for heart attacks.

Do you know your target numbers?

In Chapter 7, we gave you a list of five key numbers to know, in addition to an ideal or target range in which each number should fall. That's a good starting point, but you'll need to set your individual target numbers with your doctor, based on your unique situation. Remember that individual risk factors can influence and build off each other. For example, if your BMI is very high, your first target might be to move out of the obese category into the overweight category, or to lose 10 percent of your body weight.

Another number that needs to be individualized is your LDL cholesterol. If you're considered at very high risk of developing heart disease, your doctor may suggest you aim for an LDL level of 100 milligrams per deciliter of blood (mg/dL) or less. This might be the case if you have several risk factors, such as diabetes, metabolic syndrome or smoking. If you've been diagnosed with coronary artery disease or previously had a heart attack, your doctor may recommend a goal of 70 mg/dl or less.

Use the search tool on the Mayo Clinic Web site (www.mayoclinic.com) to locate an on-line calculator that will help you find out if your LDL level is within an optimal range.

Plans to reach your targets

Once you've established your primary risk factors, you and your doctor can prioritize and set your targets. (Remember the description of outcome goals? Think of outcome goals as your targets.) Typically, your doctor will help you establish the targets at achievable levels that will make positive impacts on your risk factors.

Your next step is identifying performance goals that help you reach your targets — these goals should be simple and practical. There's no "right" way to determine them — it depends largely on what you feel capable of and comfortable doing. But the more aligned they are with your likes and dislikes, your preferences and priorities, the greater your chance of success and enjoyment.

This may require you to make some major lifestyle changes. Hearing that, you may think, "I'll never be able to do this, so why bother?" Slow down! Take it one step at a time. You don't need to work on everything at once. Proceed at a pace with which you're comfortable.

Chances are, achieving your targets will require a combination of performance goals, whether it's diet, exercise, sleep, weight loss, medications or something more. Alongside your targets, list the performance goals that you think will help you achieve each target. Here are some examples:

Targets	Performance goals
BMI in a healthy range	▸ Eat a balanced diet. ▸ Limit sweets and fatty foods. ▸ Exercise most days of the week.
Exercise 150 minutes a week	▸ Schedule time for exercise. ▸ Start with a plan for 10 minutes a day and then gradually extend the time. ▸ Set up weekly workouts with an exercise partner.
Blood pressure below 120/80	▸ Take regular readings with a home monitor. ▸ Limit salt intake to less than 1,500 mg a day. ▸ Exercise most days of the week.

If you smoke, quitting is by far the most important thing you can do to reduce heart disease risk. And for most smokers, quitting isn't a minor change. Take all the time you need to stop tobacco use before you focus on other goals. See Chapter 6 for tips.

Sometimes it helps to break down performance goals into a series of more specific, measurable actions — ones you can achieve more quickly.

For example, if you decide that a performance goal for improving your diet is to eat more vegetables and fruits, you can come up with simple actions for doing that. They may include adding fruit to your cereal, having a side salad with lunch and having fruit for dessert. All of these actions can help you achieve your performance goal.

It's a good idea to regularly track your progress with performance goals — you can do so with the help of a daily or weekly checklist. Continue to update your doctor on how you're doing and when problems arise. The more you can stay focused on the small, achievable actions, the better your chances are of achieving your targets.

Do's and don'ts of goal setting

Goals are meant to inspire you, not make you feel like a failure if you don't meet them. Try these suggestions to avoid common missteps.

Do:

+ Write down your goals and track your progress over time.

+ Cast your goals in a positive light — avoid the "no" mentality. Rather than, "I won't snack on any more junk food," how about "I'll keep fruit or a few nuts handy if I'm hungry between meals."

+ Each day, write down a goal that you can take action on during the day. Keep it handy and read it often.

+ Fine-tune a goal if you've tried for a while and find it too challenging. But don't change your goal simply out of convenience.

+ Celebrate your success along the way. Reward yourself, whether it's a simple neck massage, an hour to yourself, or a new music or movie download.

Don't:

+ Neglect enjoyment. It's key to find satisfaction in the changes you're making.

+ Base your goals on what someone else thinks you should do — make sure your goals are your own.

+ Get caught in the terrible "toos" — trying to do too much, too soon, too hard. Keep a realistic perspective. Start out in small steps.

+ Look too far ahead, or berate yourself about the past. It's what you do today that will help you meet your goal.

+ Give up if you're feeling discouraged. Everyone fails once in a while — just get back up and don't lose sight of your goals.

CHAPTER 10

TAKE YOUR MEDICATIONS

There's a vast array of medications you can take to improve heart health, but that's not the focus of this chapter. The key word in the chapter title is the verb "take." A common challenge for anyone living with heart disease is taking medications regularly as prescribed.

? TRUE OR FALSE

If you have had a heart attack, taking a daily aspirin can reduce your risk of having another heart attack.

- True
- False

True. If you have had a heart attack, taking daily aspirin decreases your chance of another heart attack. If you have never had a heart attack, talk to your doctor to find out if aspirin is right for you.

You benefit from eating healthier, moving more and sleeping better. But these changes may accomplish only so much. Medications also may be necessary to prevent or manage heart disease. This is especially true for underlying medical conditions that lifestyle changes alone can't modify sufficiently. Different medications can improve heart function, lower cholesterol, and treat high blood pressure, heart failure or atrial fibrillation.

The goal is to take your medicines correctly and consistently for as long as you need them — and with heart drugs, that often means the rest of your life. If you stop taking your medications, your condition may worsen or your symptoms may return. If you don't take your medications as directed, they may not work, or they could cause harmful side effects.

So, why do so many people struggle to take their medications as their doctors have ordered?

I can DO this!

I'll build each step of my Healthy Heart Plan week by week with these simple goals:

+ Make a list of all the medications I take, including doses and when I need to take them. I'll store a copy of my list in a safe place in case of emergencies.

+ Learn the reasons why I'm taking each of my medications.

+ Discuss with my doctor any herbal and dietary supplements and over-the-counter medications I'm taking to make sure they don't have serious side effects or interact with my prescription medications.

Understanding the problem

There are many reasons why people have problems staying on track when they take medications. For starters, almost everyone forgets to take his or her pills from time to time.

But there are other reasons why people may struggle. Many don't like the side effects of a drug or just don't like taking medicine, period. Others feel overwhelmed when they're taking too many medications or they don't understand how or when to take them.

Some people don't notice any changes, so they stop taking a drug. The opposite can happen: People start feeling better, so they stop taking a drug. The high cost of drugs also is an issue.

You're more likely to take all your medications correctly if you understand why you take them and you develop routines for when and how to take them. Getting at least some answers to the following questions about each medicine you take will help:

- What is the brand name and generic name of this medication?
- Can I get a less expensive version?
- What is the reason for taking it?
- What happens if I don't take it?
- What time of day should I take it?
- How do I take it — with food or on an empty stomach? Can it be chewed or crushed, or must it be swallowed?
- How many pills do I take, and how often do I take them?
- How long will I need to take the drug?
- Should I avoid certain activities, foods or beverages when taking the drug?
- Are there other medications, vitamins or supplements I should avoid when taking the drug?
- What should I do if I miss a dose?
- How often do I need refills?
- What are the risks and side effects?
- What do I do if I have side effects?
- How do I know if the medication is working?
- Is it safe to use during pregnancy or breast-feeding?

You may request written information about each medication from your doctor or pharmacist. Be sure your doctor knows about all of the medications you take, including other prescriptions, over-the-counter medicines, vitamins, and herbal or dietary supplements.

Can daily aspirin prevent heart disease?

Has your spouse been nagging you to take a daily aspirin to prevent heart disease? Aspirin gets a lot of attention, but who should be taking it? The answer may be more complicated than you think.

While a daily low-dose aspirin may lower your risk of heart disease, heart attack and stroke, it's not the right choice for everyone, and it can be dangerous for some people. Aspirin interferes with your blood's clotting action, so it helps prevent blood clots that can cause a heart attack. But daily use of aspirin can have serious side effects, including internal bleeding.

If you've had a heart attack, aspirin has likely already been prescribed by your doctor because it can help prevent a second heart attack. Lifelong aspirin is also recommended for anyone who's had a procedure to place a stent in a coronary artery. In either case, you should not stop taking aspirin without consulting your doctor — stopping aspirin can increase your risk of a heart attack. If you've had a stroke, taking an aspirin reduces your risk of having another stroke.

However, if you've never had a heart attack or stroke, the question of whether to take aspirin is controversial, and recommendations may change.

Bottom line: Talk to your doctor before starting daily aspirin therapy — or, if it's already been prescribed, before stopping it.

> " It was hard to be patient and stick with my medications but they worked!"

Name: Brenda

Event: Brenda went to the hospital complaining of severe shortness of breath. She was diagnosed with heart failure. "I was so scared, because if medications did not work, I would need a heart transplant."

Outcome: Brenda takes several medications to strengthen her heart and control fluid buildup. She's also changed her lifestyle radically — she lost weight, is eating right and exercising regularly, and watching her salt and fluid intake. Her heart, which had been over twice its size and barely pumping, is almost normal now. "I have a lot more energy for my family," she says. "I was pretty much a couch potato before, but now I can play with my kids."

Overcoming the challenges

Every drug has specific benefits, side effects and rules for use. These tips can help you overcome the challenges.

Challenge: Difficulty remembering to take medications

+ Take your drugs at the same time every day. Connect pill taking to other daily habits, such as before meals or after teeth brushing.

+ Set your phone or watch alarm to signal the time, or use a free service that will send you email or text message reminders.

+ Hang up reminder notes on the bathroom mirror or refrigerator.

+ Ask a friend to remind you. If your friend takes medications, use a buddy system to call each other every day.

+ Write your schedule on a calendar or dry-erase board, and check the day off afterward.

Challenge: Unpleasant side effects

+ Know what symptoms to watch for.

+ Discuss with your doctor to see if your prescription can be adjusted.

Challenge: Dislike of medications or belief they're not needed

+ Find out how each medication works and how it helps you.

+ Ask your doctor what might happen if you don't take the medication.

Challenge: Too many medications

+ Organize your pills in a pillbox at the beginning of each week.

+ Ask your doctor about ways to reduce the number of drugs.

Challenge: Uncertainty taking a medication

+ Use a coding system to mark bottles with a different color for different times of the day.

+ Keep a folder with printed materials about each type of medication.

Challenge: Too expensive

+ Ask your doctor if a lower cost or generic version is available.

+ Check on programs that offer financial help, for example, the Partnership for Prescription Assistance: www.pparx.org.

If you're depressed ...

An issue that can sidetrack your ability to stay on track with medications is depression, a condition that's common among people with heart disease. Being even mildly depressed can double the chance you won't take your medications. If you're feeling down or hopeless, or finding little interest in life, talk to your doctor about whether you might have depression.

+ Don't split tablets unless your doctor OKs it.

+ Don't share pills with friends.

Challenge: Travel, illness or change in routine

+ Plan ahead for how and when you'll refill prescriptions.

+ Stay on top of your medications when your routine changes — which is likely to happen whenever you travel.

+ Carry an adequate supply of medications. Ask your pharmacist if you can get a weekly travel pack made.

Common heart medications

Angiotensin-converting enzyme (ACE) inhibitors help lower blood pressure and improve the heart's pumping action. People with high blood pressure who can't take ACE inhibitors may take drugs called angiotensin II receptor blockers (ARBs).

Anticoagulants and anti-platelets help prevent blood clots from forming in your blood vessels or heart. People who have chest pain (angina), had a heart attack, have atrial fibrillation, or have stents or mechanical heart valves in place usually take these medications.

Beta blockers slow the heart rate and lower blood pressure, and are used to treat angina, high blood pressure, heart failure and some heart rhythm disorders.

Calcium channel blockers relax blood vessels and are used to treat high blood pressure, angina and some heart rhythm disorders.

Water pills (diuretics) keep fluid from collecting in the body and reduce swelling in the legs and ankles. They're used to treat high blood pressure and heart failure.

Nitrates relieve chest pain by relaxing blood vessels.

Statins lower cholesterol.

Side effects and interactions

The list of medications used to treat heart disease is a long one. Any of the drugs may cause side effects, ranging from coughs and rashes to headaches, dizziness and internal bleeding. Some heart medications may also interact with foods, beverages, dietary supplements and other drugs you take in dangerous ways.

The more medications you take, the greater your chances of unwanted side effects or interactions. To help ensure that you're taking your drugs safely:

+ Read all drug labels carefully.

+ Review all medications you take with your doctor to check for possible harmful interactions.

+ Ask what you need to avoid — foods, beverages, over-the-counter drugs — when taking your medications.

+ Contact your doctor about any new symptom you notice after taking a medication.

+ Keep a record of all medications and supplements. Identification is easier when you keep them in their original containers.

+ If your medication is prescribed for a certain amount of time, make sure to take all doses until the prescription is complete.

+ Find out if you need blood tests or other tests to help monitor the effects of your medications.

+ If you're pregnant or planning a pregnancy, ask your doctor about medications. Some are risky during pregnancy and breast-feeding.

+ Never stop taking a medication or change the dosage without consulting your doctor first.

+ Know when to call your doctor or seek emergency help.

Are statins safe?

If you have high cholesterol, your doctor may recommend taking medications called statins to lower total cholesterol and reduce your risk of a heart attack or stroke. Most people on statins will take them for the rest of their lives. Some people have statin side effects — the most common are muscle aches, pain and weakness. Don't stop taking your statin medication for any period of time without talking to your doctor first. Your doctor may be able to come up with an alternative treatment plan that can help you lower your cholesterol without uncomfortable side effects.

To relieve statin side effects, your doctor may recommend:

+ Taking a break from statin therapy to see if your aches and pains are due to statins

+ Changing the type or dosage of statin you're taking

+ Taking other cholesterol-lowering drugs instead of statins

+ Using coenzyme Q10 supplements or other natural substances, such as fish oil, red yeast rice or soluble fiber, such as oat bran

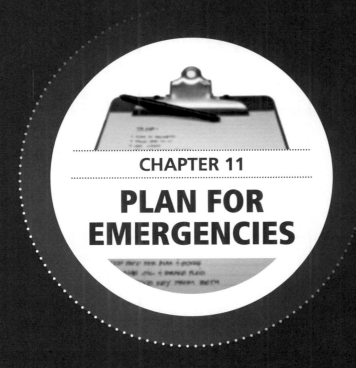

CHAPTER 11

PLAN FOR EMERGENCIES

Just as you might plan for what to do in case of fire, knowing what to do if you or someone else faces a cardiac emergency can make a life or death difference.

(?) TRUE OR FALSE

If you witness someone who collapses and is unresponsive, you should call 911, give two breaths, and then start chest compressions.

● True
● False

False. Mouth to mouth breathing is not necessary for bystander CPR. Call 911 and start chest compressions.

Whether you've been diagnosed with heart disease or not, it makes sense for you to be prepared for a heart attack or other heart-related emergency. In the United States, about 300,000 people die each year when their hearts stop before they make it to the hospital, or while they're in the emergency room. Many of those deaths could have been prevented through fast action.

A quick response to an emergency is much easier if you've had a chance to think through in advance what to do if you or someone else experiences alarming symptoms. Consider what you'd do if this happens at home or at work, if you're traveling, or if it occurs in the middle of the night.

Prepare a response plan for heart-related emergencies, including contact numbers. Share it with your family. With a plan in place, you'll save time in case of an emergency and may help save a life.

I can DO this!

I'll build each step of my Healthy Heart Plan week by week with these simple goals:

+ Memorize the signs and symptoms of a heart attack.

+ Know what to do for someone who's having cardiac arrest. Consider taking a course in cardiopulmonary resuscitation (CPR) through the American Heart Association or the American Red Cross.

+ Create a plan for responding to heart-related emergencies I will share with my family members and close friends.

5 keys for emergencies

Use these keys to plan for the worst —
while hoping for the best, and doing
everything to reduce your risk of ever
needing these plans.

1 **Recognize the warning signs.**
Your first step is to recognize
the warning signs of a heart-related
emergency. That may sound obvious,
but most Americans don't know the
signs and symptoms of a heart attack.
It's not like in a Hollywood movie,
where you clutch your hand to your
chest and fall down. Heart attacks
typically start slowly, with mild pain.

Heart attack emergency. Chest pain is
the classic symptom, but it often doesn't
feel the way people expect. Rather
than intense, sudden pain, it may start
gradually and feel like uncomfortable
pressure in the center of the chest. The
discomfort lasts for a few minutes or
goes away and comes back.

- Chest discomfort
- Discomfort or pain in your jaw,
  neck, back, arms or stomach
- Shortness of breath
- Weakness, lightheadedness or loss
  of consciousness

- Cold sweat
- Nausea or vomiting

High blood pressure emergency.
Extremely high blood pressure can
cause an emergency. Without treatment, the crisis can lead to a stroke,
heart attack and other life-threatening
problems.

- Chest pain
- Shortness of breath
- Back pain
- Numbness or weakness
- Change in vision
- Difficulty speaking

Heart failure emergency. Heart
failure can cause a sudden, life-threatening buildup of fluid in the lungs.

- Trouble breathing or a feeling of
  suffocating
- Bubbly, wheezing or gasping sound
  when you breathe
- Pink, frothy sputum when you cough
- Breathing difficulty along with
  profuse sweating
- Blue or gray tone to your skin
- Severe drop in blood pressure
  resulting in lightheadedness, dizziness, weakness or fainting

Ask your doctor if there are other emergency symptoms you should be aware of, and if there's information, such as a list of your medications, you'd need to have on hand in case you're rushed to the hospital.

2 Delay is deadly. If you notice signs and symptoms that could signal a heart emergency, act immediately by calling 911 or emergency help. Don't drive to the hospital or have a family member or friend take you unless that's your only option.

Even if you're not sure it's a heart attack, whenever something feels different, get it checked out. The first hour of a heart attack is the most dangerous because an irregular heart rhythm may develop, leading to sudden cardiac arrest.

In addition, treatment is most effective when it's given within an hour of the start of signs and symptoms. Even if your heart stops beating, emergency personnel often can deliver a life-saving shock to restart the heart.

Unfortunately, many people wait too long to seek medical help — half of all

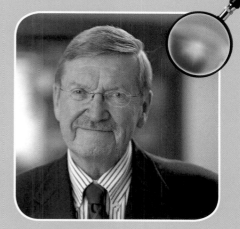

Specialist focus:

Roger D. White, M.D., is an expert in anesthesiology at Mayo Clinic.

Bystanders often do nothing when a person loses responsiveness but may still be attempting to breathe. The gasping lasts a short time, but it's a critical time because the heart has stopped beating. That is already cardiac arrest. Call 911 and begin chest compressions immediately.

heart attack victims wait two hours or more before going to the emergency room. They may put off getting help because they don't recognize the symptoms, don't want to bother others, are embarrassed about causing a scene, or worry that their symptoms are a false alarm. Some people are afraid to admit that the symptoms could be serious, or they think they're caused by something else.

3 **Start CPR if someone's in trouble.** Anyone can help save a life, even if you haven't been trained in cardiopulmonary resuscitation (CPR). A new hands-only CPR technique is easy to learn and can dramatically improve the chances of survival. If you see an adult collapse suddenly, here's what you can do:

+ Check to see if the person is conscious. If the person appears unconscious, see if he or she is responsive to your voice ("Are you OK?") and to tapping on the shoulder. If the person doesn't respond, call 911 or send someone to do it.

+ Roll the person onto his or her back. Kneel beside the person, next to the neck and shoulders.

+ Prepare to start chest compressions. Place your hands, one on top of the other, over the center of the

Hands-only CPR
Put the heel of one hand on the center of the chest, over the sternum. Lace your hands together, one on top of the other, with your shoulders directly over your hands.

chest. Keep elbows straight and shoulders directly over your hands.

+ Push hard and fast, compressing the chest at least two inches. Use your body weight as you push straight down. Let the chest rise without taking your hands off the chest. Push at a rate of 100 or more compressions a minute.

+ Keep repeating these actions without interruption until medical help arrives, or the person shows obvious signs of recovery. If you tire and someone else is nearby, ask that person to take over, keeping interruptions to a minimum.

Conventional CPR combines chest compressions with mouth-to-mouth breathing. If you're trained in conventional CPR and are confident in its use, you should follow that technique.

Hands-only CPR simplifies the process if you're not trained in conventional CPR or are uncomfortable with mouth-to-mouth contact. It's been shown to be just as effective as conventional CPR during the first few minutes of a cardiac emergency.

911 Sudden cardiac arrest

Sudden cardiac arrest isn't the same as a heart attack. A heart attack occurs when blood supply to the heart is cut off. In cardiac arrest, electrical impulses in the heart are chaotic, rapid or cease altogether, causing the heart to stop beating. Immediate CPR is critical to treating cardiac arrest.

Don't use hands-only CPR for:

✔ Infants and children under age 8
✔ People who collapsed because of breathing problems, a drug overdose or drowning
✔ Someone you find already unconscious and not breathing

In these cases, the person would likely benefit more from conventional CPR.

The point is: Be prepared. The chance of survival for a person who goes into cardiac arrest can double or triple if a bystander starts CPR before emergency medical services arrive.

> " Very few people who go through what I went through ever make it."

Name: Howard

Event: One cold winter evening, Howard, a 54-year-old chef, headed to the grocery store. He experienced cardiac arrest just outside the store and fell to the sidewalk.

Outcome: Volunteer first responders and emergency personnel took turns performing a marathon of CPR and shocks from a defibrillator for 96 minutes — 30 minutes longer than any other previously documented case of out-of-hospital cardiac arrest. "After surviving this, I'm still trying to figure out what my purpose is," says Howard. "I know I want to help whomever I can, and to do something meaningful. Hopefully, telling my story will give a new jolt to CPR."

④ Use defibrillation, if necessary. CPR can be a vital step in the lifesaving process and can keep some blood flowing to the heart and brain for a short time. But if your heartbeat becomes dangerously fast or chaotic — possibly putting your life in danger — the only way to restore normal rhythm is with defibrillation.

You may have seen this procedure if you've watched medical shows on television, when a person is shocked back to life by a doctor who yells "clear," then delivers one or more jolts of electricity to the chest.

An automatic external defibrillator (AED) is a small, portable device that senses your heart's rhythm. If it senses an abnormal rhythm that's correctable, it delivers an electric jolt that resets your heart back to a normal rhythm, possibly saving your life. However, an AED works only for specific types of rhythm problems.

In addition to being carried by police and ambulance crews, AEDs are commonly available in many public places, including malls, office buildings, sports arenas, golf courses, airports, and community or senior citizen centers.

You don't need special training to use AEDs. They come with instructions and provide real-time, step-by-step voice prompts that guide you through the process.

If you have to use an AED on someone, it's critical that you call 911 or local emergency services first. Begin CPR before you turn on the AED to use it. You may need to restart CPR again after a shock is delivered if the person remains unresponsive.

AEDs are available without a prescription for use at home. But first talk to your doctor about the pros and cons of owning one. For most people who are at high risk of sudden cardiac death, doctors will recommend an implantable cardioverter-defibrillator (ICD) rather than an AED.

5 **Involve your family.** If something should happen to you, do family members know what to do? Here are tips to enlist their support:

+ Talk with them about the warning signs of a heart attack and the importance of immediately calling for medical help.

CPR training

Check with the American Heart Association or the American Red Cross for how to find CPR classes and online courses at:
www.heart.org
www.handsonlycpr.org
www.redcross.org

+ Explain that family members should call 911 or local emergency services rather than attempting to drive you to the hospital.

+ Arrange in advance who would care for your children or other dependents in an emergency. Emergency medical personnel typically contact a relative or friend to make emergency arrangements for your dependents.

+ Consider making a written heart attack survival plan and keeping a copy in your wallet or purse. The plan should include vital medical information, such as the medications you take, any allergies, your doctor's contact information and a person to contact in case of emergency.

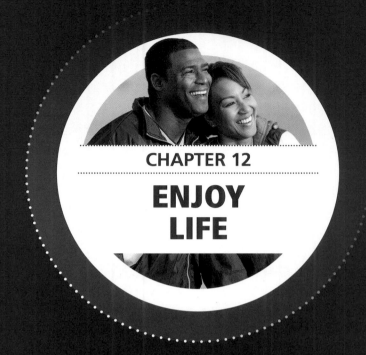

CHAPTER 12

ENJOY LIFE

A healthy life isn't just about getting all the numbers right. It's also about relaxation and fun, love and laughter. Discover what brings you joy and satisfaction.

(?) TRUE OR FALSE

Frequent episodes of intense anger increase the risk of heart attack.
- True
- False

True. Studies have shown that intense and unresolved anger increases the risk of heart attack. The good news: Laughing has been found to be beneficial for your heart.

You can track how many servings of vegetables and fruits you eat, how many minutes you exercise, and how many hours you sleep. It's harder to put a number on relaxation. Ideally, all the activities you do for your heart health should be enjoyable for you — your healthy heart plan isn't intended as a punishment or "life sentence." In fact, enjoying life is an important key to heart health.

Just as your genetic makeup, physical fitness and lifestyle habits influence your heart health, so do your mental and emotional states. Distrust, hostility, chronic stress, pessimism, hopelessness and lack of social connection have all been linked to heart problems. On the flip side, optimism, caring, social support and humor may lower your risk of heart disease and death.

You can't expect to change everything about your life for the better. But you can use happiness and satisfaction to bolster your self-image, buffer the impact of stressful events and keep nagging problems in perspective.

I can DO this!

I'll build each step of my Healthy Heart Plan week by week with these simple goals:

+ Take 10 minutes for myself each day to do something I enjoy, such as reading, working on a hobby or listening to music.

+ Find an opportunity to volunteer in my community, even if it's only a couple of hours on a weekend.

+ Get in touch with friends — call, email or meet for a walk or a meal.

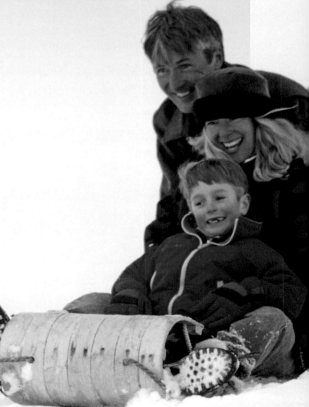

5 keys to enjoying life

It's not as easy as flipping on a switch, but you can learn to be happier — to feel more connected and less stressed, to maintain an optimistic outlook.

1 **Build a social support network.** For many people, relationships provide the strongest meaning and purpose in life. Social support — the emotional comfort and practical help you get from family, friends, colleagues and community — not only gives you a sense of belonging, self-worth and security, but also can help you stay well.

People with strong support networks are less likely to develop heart disease than are people with poor social support. If you have a heart attack, support can improve recovery and quality of life, especially for women.

These suggestions may help strengthen your support network:

+ **Volunteer.** Join a cause that's important to you. You'll meet people who share similar interests and values. Giving to others may lower your stress level and reduce your risk of heart problems.

+ **Join a club.** Check out the local community center, yoga studio, or hiking or cycling club. Start a walking group — you'll make friends as you exercise.

+ **Take a class.** Enrolling in a class or workshop through a local college or community center puts you in contact with others who share similar interests or pursuits.

+ **Participate in a faith community.** Many places of worship offer weekly discussion or support groups.

+ **Look online.** Social networking can help you stay connected with friends and family. Be sure to stick to reputable sites, and be cautious about arranging in-person meetings.

Make relationships with family and friends a priority. The more you invest in relationships, the more willing people are to provide support when you need it. Here are tips for nurturing relationships:

+ **Show appreciation.** Let family and friends know, by words as well as by actions, how important they are to you, thank them, and let them know you're glad they're part of your life. Be there when they need support.

+ **See the good in people.** Accept others as they are, without judgment. They will return the favor one day.

+ **Stay in touch.** Show you care by answering phone calls and emails and responding to invitations.

+ **Be a good listener.** Listen without offering your opinions immediately. Find out what's important to your friends. Avoid turning conversations into a contest — all they need is your sympathetic ear.

+ **Don't overdo it.** Be careful not to overwhelm family and friends with phone calls and emails. Save those high-demand times for when you really need them.

+ **Surround yourself with support.** Be around people who are positive and leading a healthy lifestyle. Steer clear of people who drain your energy, are constantly negative, or take part in unhealthy behaviors, such as alcohol or substance abuse.

2 **Relax and have fun.** Whether you're busy and multi-tasking or feeling bored and unproductive, devote time each day to relaxation and enjoyment. If you can, relax for at least 15 to 30 minutes every day, but even a five-minute break is rejuvenating.

+ **Schedule time for leisure.** Don't feel guilty about relaxation — it's a way to combat stress and stay healthy. Read, garden, listen to music, take a bath, socialize, or play games with family or friends.

+ **Practice relaxation techniques.** Techniques such as meditation, yoga, tai chi, massage, deep breathing and guided imagery create a positive response that counteracts the effects of stress. As with any other skill, relaxation takes practice to learn and master. Select something you enjoy and stick with it.

+ **Laugh.** Having a sense of humor feels good, relieves tension and gives your immune system a boost. Spend time with people who make you laugh. See a funny movie or share jokes. Even if it feels forced at first, practice laughing.

Specialist focus:

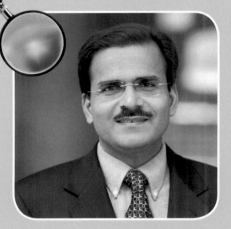

Amit Sood, M.D., is an expert in internal medicine and complementary and integrative medicine at Mayo Clinic.

Relaxation can boost heart health in a variety of ways. Biologically, relaxation decreases the stress load placed on the heart by curbing the fight-or-flight response. Taking time to relax also helps improve sleep, and it may make you less likely to eat or drink too much or engage in other unhealthy behaviors. Finally, relaxation helps people engage in more meaningful relationships, a key to heart health.

+ **Get a pet.** Animal companionship can be good for body and soul. Petting a cat, playing with a dog or listening to songbirds can be relaxing and enjoyable.

3 Reduce stress. Stress comes with living. Some stress can be useful or fun, as when you're preparing for a job interview or playing in a competitive game. But often daily hassles, demands and changes leave you on edge. Your body's response to stress — known as the fight-or-flight reaction — stays stuck in overdrive. Long-term stress of this kind puts you at risk of heart problems.

Although you can't completely eliminate stress from your life, you can manage its impact. Core parts of the Healthy Heart Plan — especially physical activity and sleep — provide built-in stress relief. Other strategies can help.

Identify causes of stress. Are you trying to do too much? For too many? With too little? Make a list of the top 10 challenges that trigger stress. Major life changes, such as divorce, new house, new job or death of a loved one, typically send stress levels through the roof. Other stressors include family conflicts, urgent deadlines, demanding bosses, unexpected bad news and unfamiliar social situations.

Recognize negative reactions.
Angry outbursts, excessive drinking, smoking, using drugs, overeating, not taking medications, neglecting responsibility, excessive worry, pessimism and procrastination can be negative reactions to stress. These reactions don't resolve the stress and may even make it worse.

If you have a tendency toward any of these behaviors, learn more positive ways of managing stress.

+ **Accept the things you can't change.** You're getting older, or you may have heart failure — these are facts you can't change. But you can still stay healthy and be active. You can continue to learn new things and help others.

+ **Slow down and scale back.** Pace yourself. Allow time to complete important tasks. Look for responsibilities you can cut back on or delegate to someone else. Learn to say no — it's OK not to take on every request that comes your way.

+ **Get organized.** Use lists, tables and reminders to prioritize daily tasks. Break them down into smaller steps if you have to. Keep a written schedule. Control clutter by keeping only the things you need.

+ **Plan ahead.** Think in advance about challenges that might arise, and how you'll meet them. When problems do come up, brainstorm ways to resolve them. If you think they're not going to be important in five years, be ready to move on.

+ **Cut down on information overload.** Take breaks from the many screens in your life — TV, computer, phone. Enjoy moments of quiet, uninterrupted time.

+ **Cultivate spirituality.** Whatever form your spirituality takes — religious observance, prayer, meditation, belief in a higher power — connecting to what's meaningful and feeling part of a greater whole can bring inner peace and a sense of purpose.

Get support. If an issue causes you stress, find a support group focused on that issue. If you're having trouble managing stress — or think you might have a more serious concern, such as anxiety or depression — seek professional help.

4 **Learn to be adaptable.** As the saying goes, the one constant in life is change. Learn how to adapt to changing needs and situations — from minor shifts in routine, such as going on vacation, to major setbacks, such as a new diagnosis or death in the family.

The ability to roll with the punches and adapt to stress is known as resilience, an inner strength that helps you rebound from setbacks. You may still experience anger and grief, but you keep functioning. It's not about toughing it out or going it alone. In fact, reaching out to others for support is a key component of being resilient.

Resilience won't make problems go away, but you can see past them and still find enjoyment in life. If you aren't as resilient as you'd like to be, you can develop skills to be more so.

 Dealing with lapses

You were making steady progress on your heart-healthy goals, but then you lost your resolve and slipped back into former unhealthy habits. Don't be too hard on yourself. Lapses happen, but they're temporary — just bumps in the road — and you can get back on track.

+ Don't let negative thoughts take over — mistakes happen. Consider each day a chance to start anew.

+ Clearly identify the problem, then think of possible solutions. Changing behaviors in small ways can make a big difference in your life.

+ Ask for support. Turn to others for a boost when you have difficult days.

+ Review your goals periodically to make sure they're not the problem — keep them realistic.

+ **Make every day meaningful.** Do something that gives you a sense of purpose. Don't postpone enjoyment because you're waiting for that elusive day when your life is calm and less stressful.

+ **Learn from experience.** Think back on how you've coped with hardships in the past. What were the strategies that helped you through rough times? Keep things in perspective. It's possible that what is a challenge today may be a benefit in the future.

+ **Remain hopeful.** You can't change the past, but you can look toward the future. Anticipating and accepting changes ahead may make it easier to adapt to new challenges.

+ **Be proactive.** Don't ignore problems or wish them away. Instead, figure out what needs to be done and make a plan to resolve them.

⑤ Find a realistic balance. As you focus on heart health, don't expect perfection. In this lifelong journey, you'll experience many ups and downs. If you struggle with a part of your plan — maybe you haven't been able to lose weight or you still don't like to exercise — avoid the tendency to conclude you're a failure and give up on everything.

Heart health is not an all-or-nothing proposition. You do what you can. And if it's not working, you try something else. Be realistic about what works best for you. Embrace a comfortable middle ground between doing things perfectly and doing nothing at all.

Develop the habit of optimism — always look for the positive in every situation. And learn to turn negative thoughts into positive ones. If you catch yourself thinking, "I'll never get any better," replace that thought with "There are so many things I can still do." Instead of "Everything is turning out wrong," think "I can handle the situation if I can take things one step at a time."

The process of working toward your goals brings satisfaction and a sense of purpose. With time, your new healthy behaviors will become habits. You might find that you're feeling better — and enjoying life more.

Using the Mayo Clinic Healthy Heart Plan for a lifetime

Congratulations! You've worked your way through the Mayo Clinic Healthy Heart Plan. You should now have all the essential knowledge and tools you need to help reduce your risk of heart disease and improve your heart health. This is a plan built to your specifications, based on your needs and shaped by the goals you followed from each chapter.

For now, take time to reflect on everything you've learned. You've been building your plan in distinct steps, but you're probably aware of just how closely connected and interdependent these steps are. That's exactly the point: It's the combination of steps, not individual ones, that forms a strong foundation for your heart health.

Also take time to assess how you did as you moved from step to step within the program. Which steps or goals were a little easier for you? Which steps or goals did you struggle with? Look for strategies to overcome any obstacles that may have been holding you back.

Most importantly, celebrate the fact that you've gotten this far in your quest for heart health. A key element of the plan — the "glue" that keeps everything together — is how much you enjoy what you're doing. If you like your plan and the changes it has made in your life, then you're more likely to stay committed to your goals. Never downplay the importance of enjoyment.

Looking ahead, set long-term goals for yourself. Review these goals with your doctor. Make sure the goals are ones you can achieve. And don't forget to reward yourself anytime you achieve one of your goals. Rewards are great motivators.

Charting a course for the future

My nutrition goals are:
Eat more fresh fruits and vegetab[les] and less red meat.

My activity goals are:
Watch less TV and exercise more by tak[ing] walks after dinner.

My slumber number is: 8

My smoking quit date is: January 1st

My healthy weight is: 185

My blood pressure goal is: 110/75

My cholesterol goals are:
HDL of 70 and LDL of 100

My plan to enjoy life is:
Don't sweat the small stuff, enjoy my family and friends, have the right attitude and BE HEALTHY!

✓ I have a family medical history

✓ I have a list of all my medications

✓ I know CPR

✓ I have a plan for emergencies

PART 3

IF YOU HAVE A PROBLEM

If you know how your heart works, it's easier to understand what can go wrong. That's your starting point in Part 3 — a brief, illustrated guide to the heart.

Also in this section, you'll find real-life stories of people dealing with heart disease. You'll learn that attitude and motivation may make all the difference.

CHAPTER 13

HOW YOUR HEART WORKS

You probably already know that your heart pumps blood throughout your body, but you may not know how complex its workings really are. Your heart has four separate chambers and four valves that function as one-way doors to keep blood flowing in the proper direction. Your heart has its own electrical system that triggers each heartbeat.

Your heart pumps about 5 quarts of blood in a minute, and beats about 100,000 times a day. It supplies not only its own tissues with blood, but every cell in your body through a closed network of 60,000 miles of arteries, veins and capillaries. Maintaining this blood supply to every part of your body is what makes heart health so important.

Lungs

Heart

Your heart, sitting slightly left of center in your chest, is the power source of your body's circulatory system. All the blood circulating through your body begins and ends its journey in your heart.

© MFMER

Chambers and valves

Your heart is divided into right and left sides, with a chamber on the top and bottom half of each side. The right side of your heart (colored blue on page 129) is responsible for collecting oxygen-depleted blood and waste products from your body and sending it to your lungs. The left side of your heart (colored red on page 129) receives oxygen-rich blood from your lungs and pumps it out to deliver fuel to every cell in your body. The top chambers of your heart (atria) serve as the collecting chambers before the blood moves to the lower, pumping chambers (ventricles).

Blood is supposed to move in only one direction through your heart and not go backward. Four valves — the tricuspid, mitral, pulmonary, and aortic valves — work like one-way trap doors, opening only when pushed on by blood flowing onto the next chamber. Each valve opens and closes once per heart beat, or about once every second (see insets at right).

Your heart is a muscular organ about the size of your fist. The muscles are part of a thick layer of tissue called the myocardium, which contracts and relaxes to create your heart's pumping action. The myocardium is one of the parts of your heart most often affected by disease.

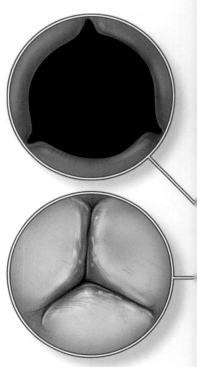

Open

Closed

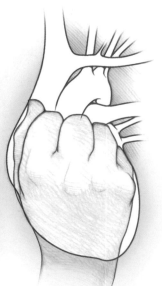

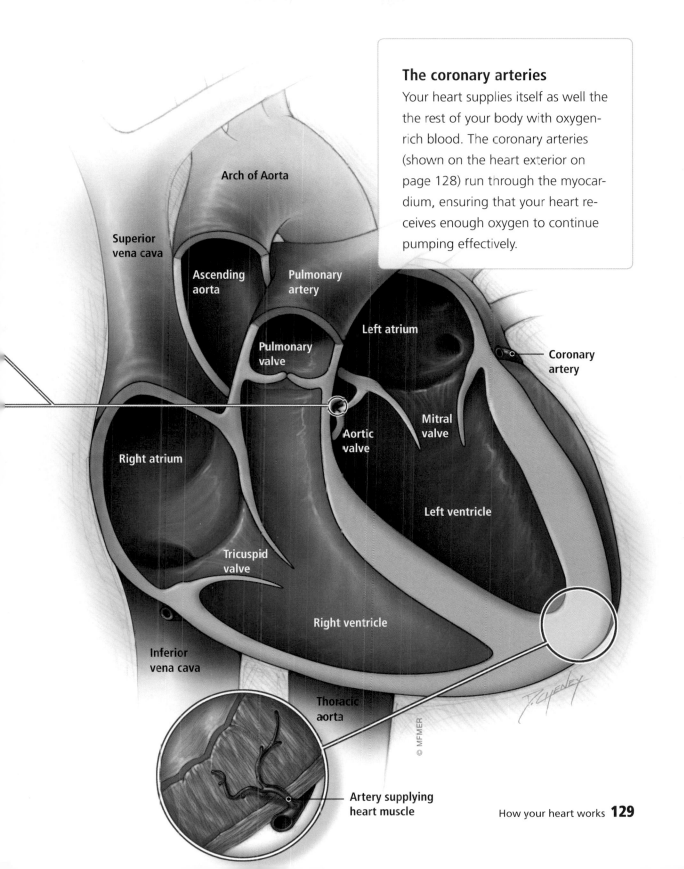

The coronary arteries

Your heart supplies itself as well the the rest of your body with oxygen-rich blood. The coronary arteries (shown on the heart exterior on page 128) run through the myocardium, ensuring that your heart receives enough oxygen to continue pumping effectively.

Arch of Aorta

Superior vena cava

Ascending aorta

Pulmonary artery

Pulmonary valve

Left atrium

Coronary artery

Aortic valve

Mitral valve

Right atrium

Left ventricle

Tricuspid valve

Inferior vena cava

Right ventricle

Thoracic aorta

Artery supplying heart muscle

© MFMER

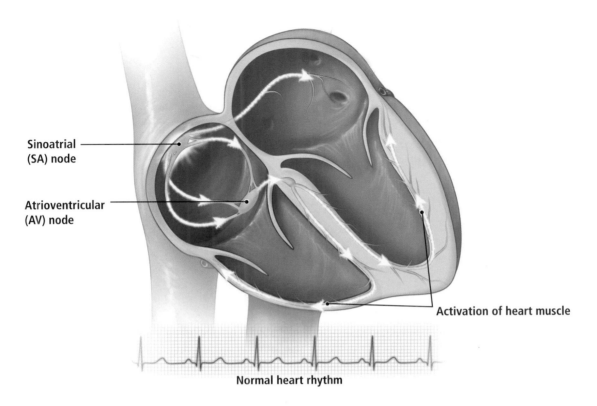

Sinoatrial
(SA) node

Atrioventricular
(AV) node

Activation of heart muscle

Normal heart rhythm

Your heartbeat

Your heart has a built-in electrical wiring system that triggers a heartbeat — a regular, coordinated cycle causing your heart's chambers to relax and contract and pump blood.

The cycle begins in the sinus node, sometimes called your heart's natural pacemaker. The sinus node is actually a group of cells located in your right atrium. The cells at the node cause an electrical impulse, which then spreads along pathways of specialized tissue in the heart to coordinate the heartbeat.

The area of the atrioventricular (AV) node collects the signals and transmits them to the two ventricles (lower chambers). The AV node is like a gatekeeper — it can slow down the heart beat if the upper chambers are beating too fast, or work as a pacemaker if the sinus node isn't functioning properly. The electrical impulses spread to the muscle of your ventricles, making your heart beat.

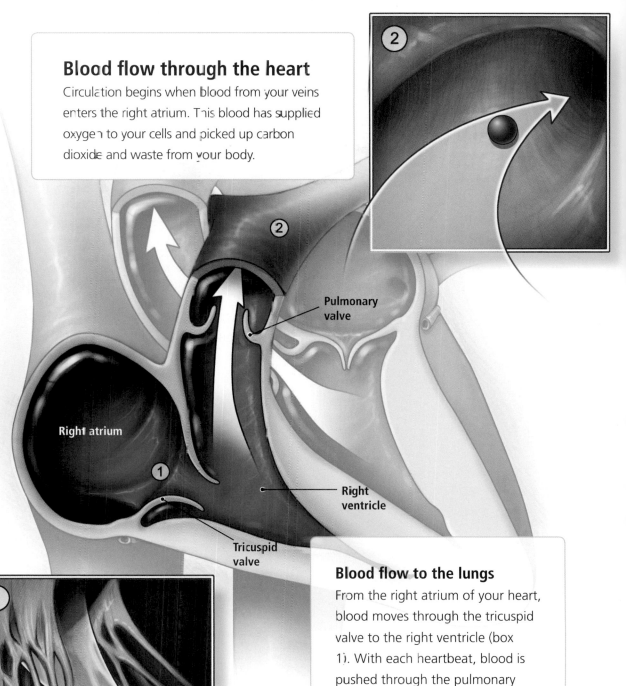

Blood flow through the heart

Circulation begins when blood from your veins enters the right atrium. This blood has supplied oxygen to your cells and picked up carbon dioxide and waste from your body.

Pulmonary valve

Right atrium

Right ventricle

Tricuspid valve

Blood flow to the lungs

From the right atrium of your heart, blood moves through the tricuspid valve to the right ventricle (box 1). With each heartbeat, blood is pushed through the pulmonary valve and travels to the lungs, where it will deposit carbon dioxide and pick up fresh oxygen (box 2).

© MFMER

Trachea

Exchange in the lungs

Blood travels through tiny blood vessels (capillaries) in your lungs. The capillaries resemble tiny webs that surround air sacs (alveoli). When you inhale, oxygen enters your windpipe (trachea) and fills the alveoli.

Dropping off waste

Carbon dioxide (CO_2), a waste product, is released through the capillaries into the alveoli and exhaled out through your windpipe.

Gas exchange in the aveoli

③

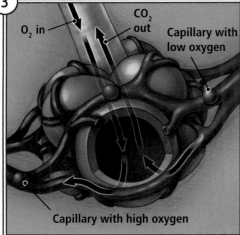

O_2 in

CO_2 out

Capillary with low oxygen

Capillary with high oxygen

③

Alveoli

Picking up oxygen

Oxygen (O_2) in the alveoli is picked up by the capillaries. Blood color turns from blue to red because it's now full of oxygen, the fuel for your body.

Low Oxygen

High Oxygen

© MFMER

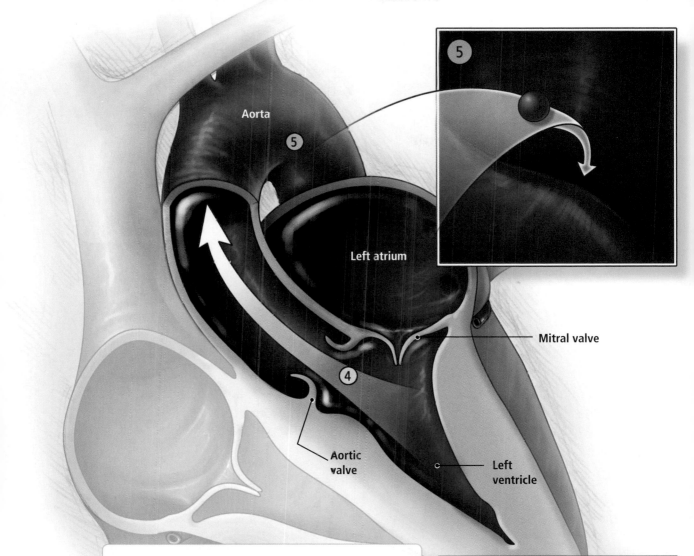

Aorta

(5)

Left atrium

Mitral valve

(4)

Aortic
valve

Left
ventricle

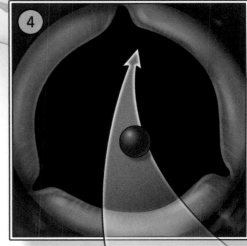

Blood flow into your body

Your blood enters the left atrium from your
lungs, then goes through the mitral valve to the
left ventricle. The ventricle pumps your blood
through the aortic valve (box 4) and into the
aorta to the rest of your body (box 5). Although
blood flow is represented here by a single cell,
your blood consists of millions of tiny cells.

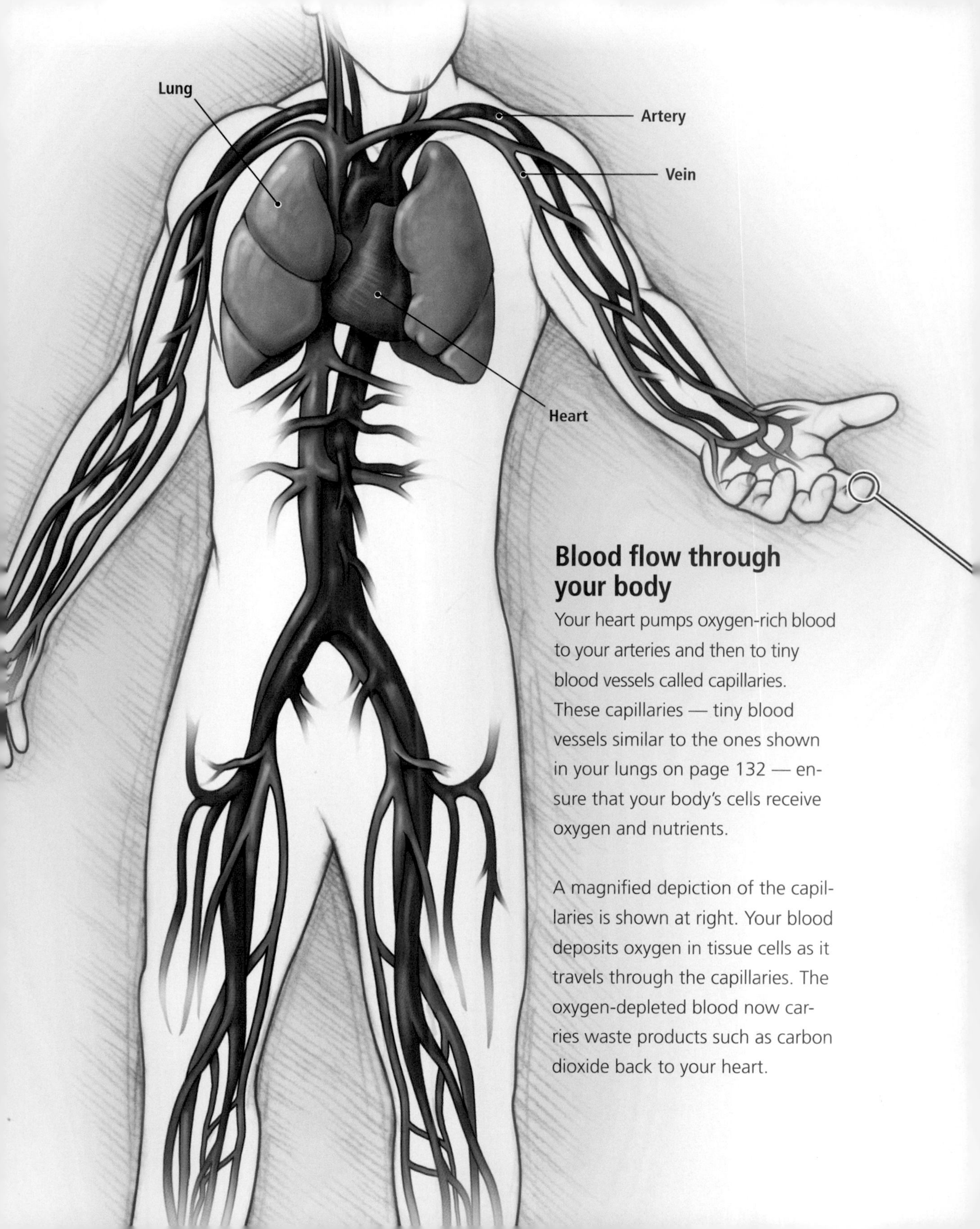

Lung

Artery

Vein

Heart

Blood flow through your body

Your heart pumps oxygen-rich blood to your arteries and then to tiny blood vessels called capillaries. These capillaries — tiny blood vessels similar to the ones shown in your lungs on page 132 — ensure that your body's cells receive oxygen and nutrients.

A magnified depiction of the capillaries is shown at right. Your blood deposits oxygen in tissue cells as it travels through the capillaries. The oxygen-depleted blood now carries waste products such as carbon dioxide back to your heart.

Back in the heart, the process begins again. Your blood is re-oxygenated and recirculated through your body.

Heart and body connection

Your heart has important connections to the rest of your body. Your brain can signal your heart to speed up or slow down, and regulate the blood pressure in your circulatory system, if necessary.

If you're in an emergency, your brain can cause your heart circulate more blood to your body, giving you a burst of energy.

The brain can signal your adrenal glands to release more hormones that speed up your heart rate.

If you have problems with your thyroid gland, your heart may speed up or slow down, affecting your heart's pumping function.

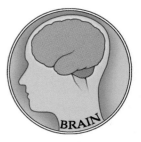

BRAIN

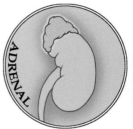

ADRENAL

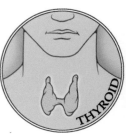

THYROID

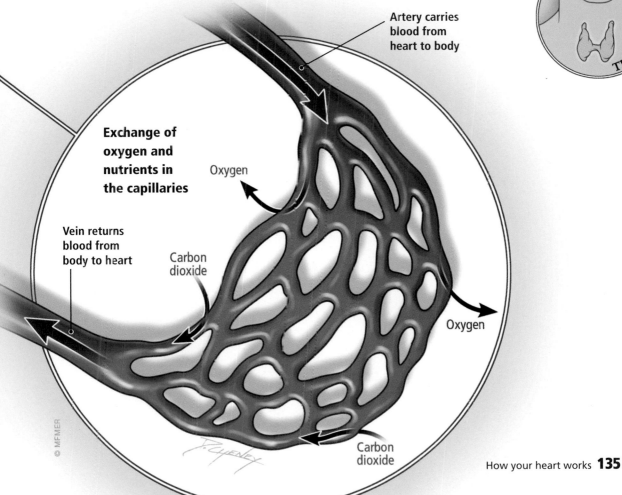

Artery carries blood from heart to body

Exchange of oxygen and nutrients in the capillaries

Oxygen

Vein returns blood from body to heart

Carbon dioxide

Oxygen

Carbon dioxide

© MFMER

CHAPTER 14

WHAT CAN GO WRONG

The flow of blood through your heart and circulatory system is an intricate process. Many things can go wrong inside and outside the heart. If blood flow is interrupted or irregular, problems can develop quickly and cascade throughout the rest of your body.

Many common forms of heart disease can eventually lead to heart failure, meaning that your heart can't pump enough blood to meet your body's needs.

Fortunately, most types of heart disease can be prevented, slowed or even reversed by following the strategies in the Mayo Clinic Healthy Heart Plan.

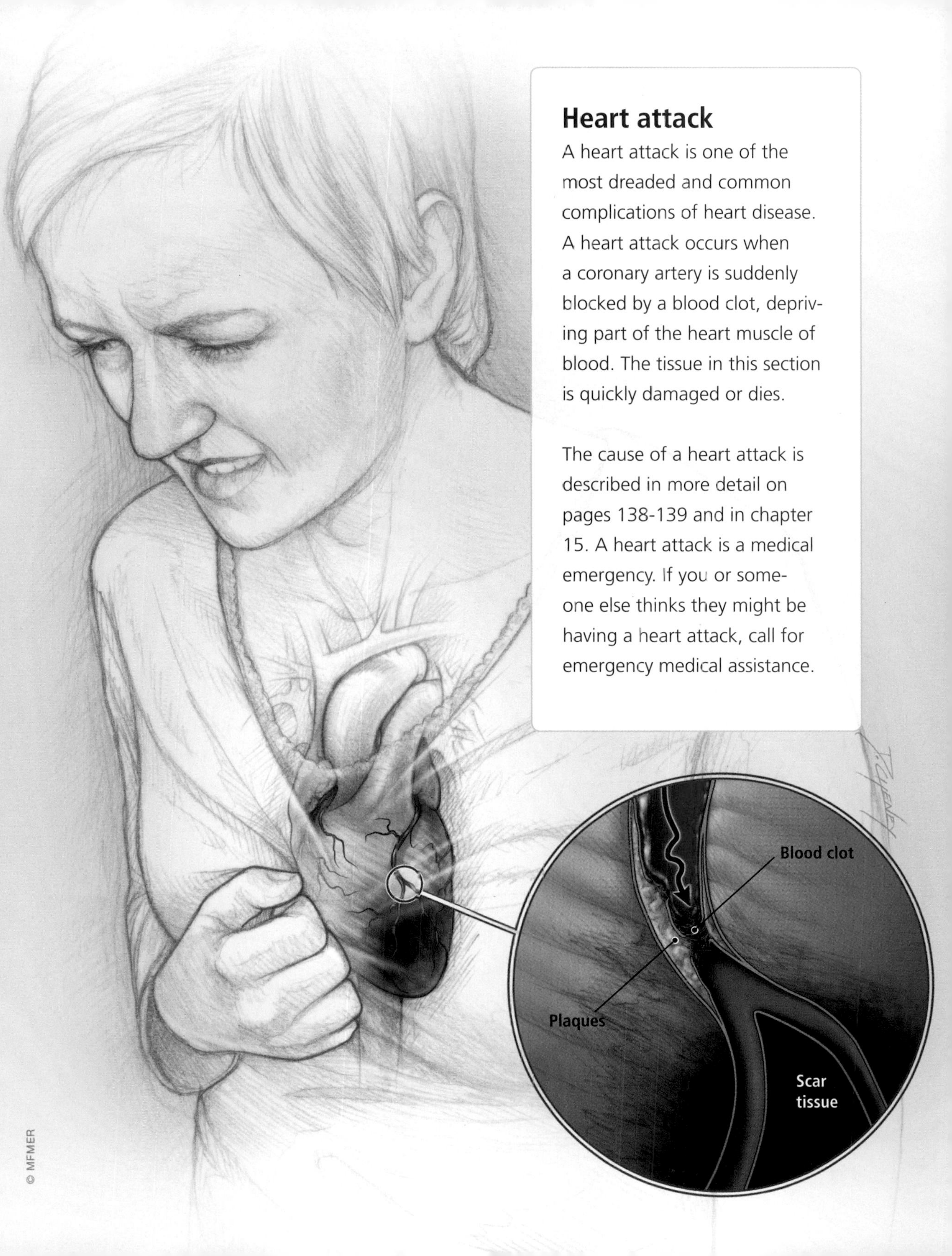

Heart attack

A heart attack is one of the most dreaded and common complications of heart disease. A heart attack occurs when a coronary artery is suddenly blocked by a blood clot, depriving part of the heart muscle of blood. The tissue in this section is quickly damaged or dies.

The cause of a heart attack is described in more detail on pages 138-139 and in chapter 15. A heart attack is a medical emergency. If you or someone else thinks they might be having a heart attack, call for emergency medical assistance.

Blood clot

Plaques

Scar tissue

© MFMER

Healthy artery

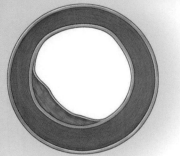

Plaques begin to form in the lining of an artery.

The artery becomes more abnormal with plaque growth.

One of these plaques may rupture.

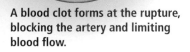

A blood clot forms at the rupture, blocking the artery and limiting blood flow.

Atherosclerosis

Atherosclerosis is a progressive narrowing of your arteries due to the buildup of fat and other substances that form plaques. Although the exact cause is unknown, atherosclerosis may start with damage or injury to an inner layer of the artery. The damage may be due to high blood pressure, high cholesterol, tobacco use, diabetes, inflammation, or other causes.

The process can happen anywhere in your body, and can lead to coronary artery disease, heart attack and stroke. Developing atherosclerosis doesn't mean you're doomed to having these conditions. It's possible to slow or reverse the process and reduce your chance of complications.

Multiple blockages
In any artery, plaques can form multiple narrowed areas (stenosis) or blockages (occlusions). These plaques limit blood flow.

Unstable plaques
Some plaques become unstable, developing cracks in the lining and rupturing, which allows fat and other substances to pour into the artery.

Diseased artery

Ruptured plaque

Dangerous clot
A blood clot forms where plaques rupture. The clot can completely block blood flow through the vessel, causing a heart attack.

© MFMER

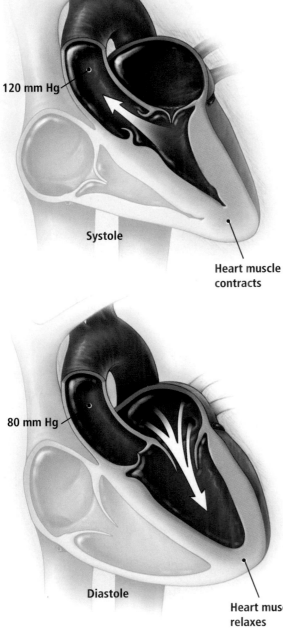

120 mm Hg

Systole

Heart muscle
contracts

80 mm Hg

Diastole

Heart muscle
relaxes

High blood pressure

Your heart and blood vessels form a closed system called the circulatory system. When your heart pumps, it generates pressure in your blood vessels to move blood through your body. When your heart relaxes, the pressure in your blood vessels decreases. The pressure created by this pumping action is your blood pressure. If the force of the blood against your artery walls is too high, it may eventually cause serious health problems such as heart disease.

Systole

In the phase of your heart's pumping action called systole, your heart contracts to push blood out of the ventricles and into the rest of your body. Your systolic blood pressure — the top number in a blood pressure reading — should be below 120 mm Hg. If it's consistently higher than 140 mm Hg, you may have high blood pressure.

Diastole

In the phase of your heart's pumping action called diastole, the muscles of your heart relax and fill with blood. Your diastolic blood pressure — the bottom number in a blood pressure reading — should be below 80 mm Hg. If it's consistently higher than 90 mm Hg, you may have high blood pressure.

The silent killer

High blood pressure can cause complications throughout your body, often occurring without symptoms. High blood pressure often develops hand-in-hand with atherosclerosis.

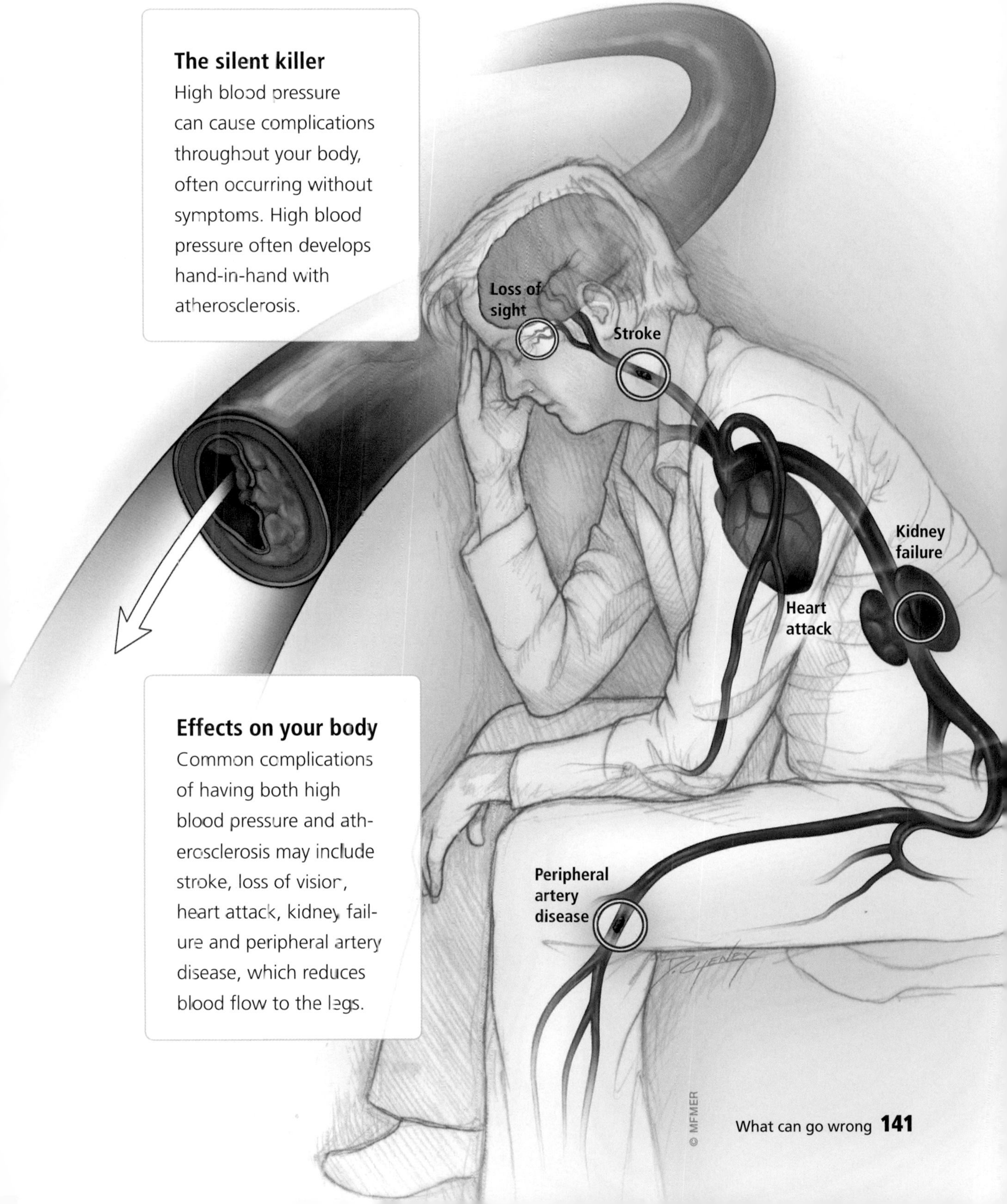

Loss of sight

Stroke

Kidney failure

Heart attack

Effects on your body

Common complications of having both high blood pressure and atherosclerosis may include stroke, loss of vision, heart attack, kidney failure and peripheral artery disease, which reduces blood flow to the legs.

Peripheral artery disease

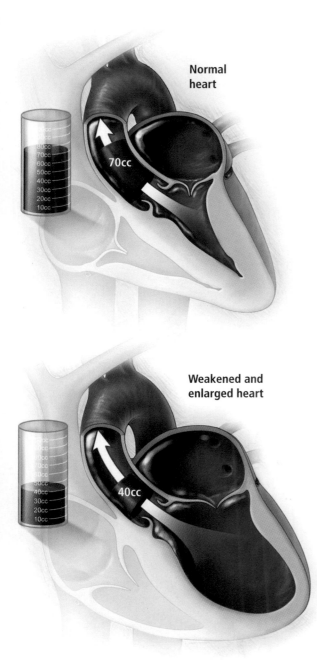

Normal heart

70cc

Weakened and enlarged heart

40cc

Heart function

Many conditions may interfere with your heart's pumping action. A normal heart (upper left) pumps out about 70 cubic centimeters (cc) of blood with every beat. The ejection fraction is the percentage of blood pumped out of the heart each time it contracts. Since the heart doesn't empty completely, the ejection fraction is never 100 percent. Instead, it's normally between 50 and 70 percent. The remaining 50 to 30 percent remains in the ventricle.

If your heart muscle weakens, it can't pump as much blood with each beat. That forces the heart to beat faster to meet your body's demands. Over time, the heart usually tries to compensate by enlarging to fill with more blood. The result (lower left) is an enlarged, weakened heart pumping a reduced amount of blood with each beat — in this example, only about 40 cc of blood.

The ejection fraction is just one measure of your heart's function. It can also be misleading. In some conditions, such as long-term high blood pressure, the heart muscle may stiffen, making it harder for your heart to fill between beats. If your heart can't fill properly, it won't pump enough blood to supply your needs — even if the ejection fraction is within the normal range.

Lung

Fluid surrounding the
lungs makes it difficult
to get a breath.

Normal
heart size

Enlarged
heart

Heart failure

Untreated heart disease of any kind and
other non-cardiac conditions such as severe
infections can make the heart too weak or
too stiff to pump effectively. When the heart
does not pump enough blood to meet your
needs, blood often backs up and causes fluid
to build up in your lungs (congest) and in
your legs, causing your legs to swell and turn
blue from lack of oxygenated blood flow
(cyanosis). This fluid in your lungs can make
you short of breath. This is worse at night
when more blood returns back to the heart.

Swollen
cyanotic
feet

© MFMER

CHAPTER 15
CORONARY ARTERY DISEASE

If your mind draws a blank when you hear "coronary artery disease," maybe this will get your attention: It's the major culprit behind heart attacks. Heart disease is the leading cause of death of both men and women in the United States, and the most common form of heart disease is coronary artery disease.

The coronary arteries provide your heart muscle with a steady supply of blood. The oxygen and nutrients in blood give your heart the energy to do its job — continuously pumping blood out to your lungs and to other parts of your body. When the arteries become damaged or blocked, partially or completely, the condition is known as coronary artery disease.

> " A nurse told me to go to the ER right away because I was having a heart attack. I thought, 'This can't be happening to me, I'm the mom, I can't be sick.' I didn't go for several hours. I had to get one son ready for prom and another off to camp. I'm lucky to be alive. "

Jeanie

Diagnosis: Coronary artery disease

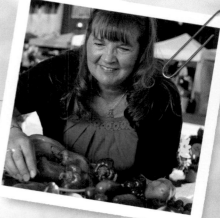

Heart event: Jeanie had been experiencing pain in both hands for weeks. A medical transcriptionist who typed for hours each week, she figured she was developing carpal tunnel syndrome. But the pain kept getting worse, moving into her arms, chest and back. Finally, she had a stress test. When she callled for the results and said she was having symptoms, nurses told her to immediately go to the hospital. But Jeanie hesitated. She wanted to talk with her teenage sons first. "I wanted to tell them what was happening because I didn't know if I would ever see them again," she says. Jeanie finally went to the hospital, where more tests showed one of the main arteries leading to her heart was almost completely blocked. She received a stent, medications and entered cardiac rehabilitation.

Outlook: "After you have a heart event, it's almost like you go through a grieving process," she says. "I had major depression. Finally I said, 'This is enough. You are going to get up and join this gym. It's going to cost you money, but you get to do something for yourself.'" Today she works out regularly, has lost weight and feels great.

Coronary artery disease (CAD) typically develops over many years. Although you may feel chest discomfort, the damage to your heart muscle may occur without any symptoms and weaken your heart's ability to pump blood. Your first sign of CAD might be a heart attack. By learning more about CAD and committing yourself to improved heart health, you can help prevent or slow the disease and reduce your risk of heart attack.

Causes

Coronary artery disease starts with small changes in the inner layer of a coronary artery, when cells become damaged or injured and stop working properly. Possible causes of this damage include smoking, high blood pressure, high cholesterol, diabetes, infections, even the aging process.

Any kind of injury in your body typically triggers inflammation. Once the inner layer of an artery is damaged, fatty deposits (plaques) tend to accumulate at the site of the injury. The plaques contain cholesterol and other substances. As plaques form, the artery wall thickens.

Deposits of plaques build up gradually, narrowing the channel and reducing blood flow (see pages 138-139). This process is called atherosclerosis. Your heart may get enough blood to fuel normal activities, but when it has to work harder — such as during exercise — it needs more blood, and the arteries can't meet the demand.

Uncommon causes of heart attack

One uncommon cause is a spasm — a brief, temporary contraction or narrowing of a coronary artery. If the spasm lasts long enough, it can cause chest pain and trigger a heart attack or a life-threatening heart rhythm disturbance. A spasm may be triggered by certain medications, use of tobacco or cocaine, or exposure to cold. Another rare cause of heart attack is a coronary artery dissection, which is a tear in a heart artery that blocks blood flow.

Treatments for CAD

Treatment for CAD starts with lifestyle changes that provide a solid foundation for heart health. It's crucial that you control high blood pressure, high cholesterol and diabetes.

Medications

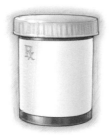

Your doctor will likely recommend aspirin to reduce blood clotting and prescribe drugs to lower cholesterol or control blood pressure. Medications to treat angina, such as nitroglycerin and beta blockers, are often prescribed. If more aggressive treatment is needed, you will likely continue taking medications.

Coronary arteries

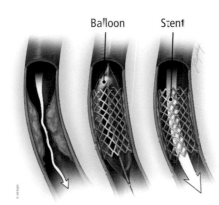

Balloon   Stent

Artery bypass

Vein bypass

Blockage

Coronary angioplasty

With this more aggressive treatment, your doctor reopens a clogged channel by inflating a tiny balloon that's inserted into the artery by a long, thin tube. Then, a small wire mesh tube (stent) is often placed to keep the channel open.

Coronary bypass

This procedure may be called for if you have severe blockage. In it, a section of healthy blood vessel is taken from another part of your body and attached above and below the blockage. This forms an alternate route for blood to flow.

Symptoms

At first, the reduced blood flow to your heart because of coronary artery disease may not cause symptoms. That's because your heart is able to increase blood flow to compensate for mildly narrowed arteries. However, as CAD becomes worse, your heart won't be able to supply enough blood to your heart muscle. Symptoms typically show up first with physical exertion and are usually relieved by rest. The classic symptom of CAD is called angina, which is pressure, tightness or discomfort in your chest or arms. Signs and symptoms of CAD, some of which are less typical (especially in women), include:

- Pressure, tightness, pain, squeezing or aching sensation in your chest or arms that may spread to neck, jaw or back
- Feeling of fullness, nausea, indigestion or heartburn

- Feeling tired or weak
- Shortness of breath
- Sweating
- Feelings of anxiety

Complications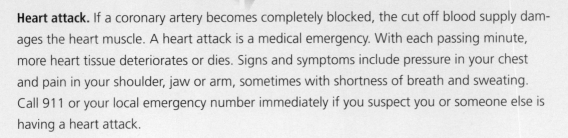

Heart attack. If a coronary artery becomes completely blocked, the cut off blood supply damages the heart muscle. A heart attack is a medical emergency. With each passing minute, more heart tissue deteriorates or dies. Signs and symptoms include pressure in your chest and pain in your shoulder, jaw or arm, sometimes with shortness of breath and sweating. Call 911 or your local emergency number immediately if you suspect you or someone else is having a heart attack.

Heart failure. If areas of your heart are chronically deprived of oxygen because of reduced blood flow, or if your heart has been damaged by a heart attack, your heart may become too weak to pump enough blood to meet your body's needs. This is known as heart failure.

Abnormal heart rhythm (arrhythmia) and sudden cardiac death. Damage to the heart muscle may cause life-threatening abnormal heart rhythms that can lead to cardiac arrest. Arrhythmias can be the first sign of a heart attack or can occur years later, due to scar formation.

Factors such as smoking, stress, heavy meals, alcohol use, excitement and exposure to cold or hot weather also can make your heart work harder.

Occasionally, plaques crack or rupture. When this happens, blood particles clump together at the site to repair the crack. The particles form a blood clot that can completely block the artery and cut off blood supply, leading to a heart attack.

Diagnosis and treatment

Your doctor can't detect a blocked coronary artery simply by listening with a stethoscope. If your family history, risk factors or symptoms suggest CAD, you may undergo one or more tests, including electrocardiography, echocardiography, stress test, CT scan, coronary angiography and nuclear scan.

Treatment for CAD starts with lifestyle changes that provide a solid foundation for heart health. It's crucial that you control high blood pressure, high cholesterol and diabetes. Your doctor will likely recommend aspirin to reduce blood clotting and prescribe drugs to lower cholesterol or control

blood pressure. Medications to treat angina, such as nitroglycerin and beta blockers, are often prescribed.

Sometimes more aggressive treatment is necessary. This is especially true if you have symptoms that aren't improving with medications, are increasing in frequency or occur while you're resting (unstable angina).

If you're having a heart attack, your doctor may order medications to dissolve the blood clots.

A coronary angioplasty procedure also may be required. Your doctor reopens a clogged channel by inflating a tiny balloon that's inserted into the artery by a long, thin tube. Then, a small wire mesh tube called a stent is often placed to keep the channel open.

If you have severe blockage in many areas or at a high-risk location, you may need a surgical procedure called coronary artery bypass. The surgeon takes a section of healthy blood vessel from another part of your body and attaches it above and below the blockage. This forms an alternate route for blood to flow around the blockage.

How can heart attacks be prevented?

You may wonder about preventive screening for coronary artery disease to try and prevent heart attacks from ever happening. With all the medical advances, why not just send people to a lab to look for plugged arteries and, when they're found, unblock the arteries with stents?

It's not as easy as it sounds. When a heart attack occurs, something has caused the plaques lining your arteries to become unstable. These plaques can rupture, which triggers the formation of a blood clot. The clot can be big enough to block the artery, causing a heart attack.

However, plaques are usually present at many locations in your coronary arteries and there's no test that can tell your doctor at which location a rupture is most likely to take place.

In addition, contrary to what you might think, many heart attacks happen in areas where not as much narrowing of your arteries has occurred rather than in areas where the most build-up of plaques is located.

Even if you've had stents placed or had coronary bypass surgery, you're not "cured." Placing a stent at one location won't prevent plaques from bursting and forming a clot somewhere else in the artery. Inserting multiple stents may not be effective because it's too difficult to determine which plaques may rupture.

Researchers are working on ways to predict which plaques are "vulnerable" to bursting and causing heart attacks. But there's so much more you can do personally. Consider this: The best defense against heart attacks and coronary artery disease is to have a good offense.

What's that mean? The most effective way to prevent heart attacks is to change your risk factors: If you smoke, stop smoking; maintain a healthy weight; eat a healthy diet; if you have diabetes or high blood pressure or high cholesterol, learn to control them; if you need medications, take them as prescribed. And get moving!

This is the stuff you've probably heard about for years. It's still true. And it works!

Women and CAD

Much of the information regarding coronary artery disease applies to both men and women. However, it's worth noting that women can face some challenges when dealing with coronary artery disease.

A big reason for this has to do with risk factors. Risk factors such as smoking, diabetes and high triglycerides appear to put women at even higher risk for CAD compared with men.

In addition, women have unique risk factors. For example, a history of complications during pregnancy (high blood pressure, diabetes and pre-eclampsia) put women at higher risk for CAD later in life.

Women are also more likely to have autoimmune conditions, such as lupus and rheumatoid arthritis, which increase their risk for CAD.

CAD is the number one killer of men and women. So, women need to recognize symptoms and be aware of their unique risk factors.

Specialist focus:

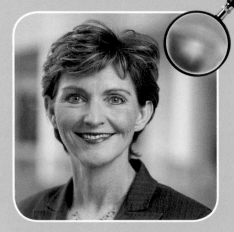

Sharonne N. Hayes, M.D., specializes in heart disease in women at Mayo Clinic.

Because CAD has been thought of as a "man's disease," many women are unaware of their risk. Women are less likely to recognize signs and symptoms of a heart attack and are less likely to call for help when they're having symptoms. They're more likely to say, "Oh, I was cooking dinner," or "I'd be embarrassed," even though they'd call 911 if someone else experienced symptoms. Once women realize their risk, they are much more likely to take heart health seriously.

Adapting the Healthy Heart Plan to CAD

Reducing your elevated risk of heart attack is a primary concern if you have coronary artery disease. Tailor the Healthy Heart Plan to your condition with the following steps.

1 Drop your LDL cholesterol level to a lower target number.
Because CAD places you at high risk of heart attack, it calls for aggressive control of your low-density lipoprotein (LDL) cholesterol level. Your doctor may recommend that you aim for a target at or below 70 milligrams per deciliter (mg/dL) — rather than the below 100 mg/dL level that's typically recommended. To reach this low target, you'll need to be fully committed to healthy eating, regular exercise and the other aspects of your plan. It's also critical to see your doctor regularly to track cholesterol levels.

2 Get into a cardiac rehabilitation program. Cardiac rehabilitation isn't just for people who've had a heart attack — anyone with coronary artery disease can benefit, especially if you've had chest pain (angina), angioplasty, stents or coronary bypass surgery. Rehabilitation typically includes education, training and support to help you live with heart disease and reduce your risk of future problems. Studies show that people who participate in cardiac rehabilitation cut their chance of dying of heart disease by nearly 30 percent and improve their symptoms.

3 Respect your medications. Many people will need to take medications long term or for the rest of their lives after being diagnosed with CAD. This can be a problem if you become bored with the routine or don't see any benefits from taking the drugs.

Remember that the drugs you're prescribed may save your life. Understand the purpose of each of your medications and create a system that keeps you on track with taking them.

Your doctor will likely recommend taking a low-dose aspirin to reduce the tendency of your blood to clot. If you've had a heart attack, aspirin can also help prevent future heart attacks. If you've had a coronary stent placed, your doctor will likely tell you to take medications to reduce the risk of blood clots forming in the stent. Aspirin is usually recommended for life along with medications such as clopidogrel

(Plavix), prasugrel (Effient) and ticagrelor (Brilinta) for up to a year or more.

Don't stop taking these blood-thinning medications without speaking to your doctor first. Stopping these medications abruptly may increase your risk of heart attack and death.

4 **Be alert for warning signs and be ready to seek help.** Understand the warning signs that signal your disease is worsening and a heart attack is more likely:

- ✔ Chest pressure, discomfort or pain that lasts more than a few minutes or goes away and comes back
- ✔ Pain extending beyond your chest to your shoulder, arm, back, or even to your teeth and jaw
- ✔ Shortness of breath
- ✔ Chest pressure that occurs at rest or more often than previous episodes
- ✔ Impending sense of doom
- ✔ Fainting
- ✔ Nausea, vomiting, prolonged heartburn or intense sweating.

Call 911 immediately if you experience these symptoms.

5 **Ask your doctor if you need a heart device.** Damage to your heart muscle from CAD may put you at risk of a life-threatening heart rhythm problem. An implantable cardioverter-defibrillator (ICD) is a small electronic device that works as a pacemaker to ensure that your heart beats in a normal rhythm. The device can also deliver a mild electrical shock if a dangerous abnormal heart rhythm persists.

→ **Additional resources:**

Mayo Clinic
www.mayoclinic.com

American Heart Association
www.heart.org

National Heart, Lung, and Blood Institute
www.nhlbi.nih.gov

A doctor who's been there

Mayo Clinic endocrinologist Bryan McIver, Ph.D., treats many people with thyroid cancer, who are facing the uncertainty and fear that comes with a potentially life-threatening illness. And he can relate to their feelings.

"There's something about having been in that position, close to the edge, that opens your eyes to what patients go through," Dr. McIver says. "Once in a while, when someone is in a particularly tough place, I'll share my story."

That story happened more than a decade ago, when Dr. McIver was 37 years old and completing his fellowship at Mayo Clinic in Rochester, Minnesota. One evening, his wife was out of town, and he arranged to meet friends for dinner. "During all of that day leading up to the dinner, I had a kind of niggling discomfort," the doctor recalls. "It wasn't really a pain, just discomfort."

Worried that he might be having a heart attack, he put himself through an informal stress test by running up seven flights of stairs. The discomfort went away, so he dismissed his concerns. After dinner, however, he experienced what felt like indigestion and took heartburn medication. On the way home, he decided to stop at his research lab. "I remember walking down that corridor and feeling unwell," he says. "No pain, just an overwhelming sense that something awful was about to happen. And that's the last I remember."

As he found out later, a nurse coming off her shift at the nearby hospital emergency room (ER) witnessed Dr. McIver fall to the floor. She checked his pulse, called for help and began CPR. A doctor heard her and helped transport Dr. McIver to the emergency room. By then, he was in complete cardiac arrest — his heart had stopped beating. The ER team was able to shock his heart back to life, but it was touch-and-go all night. He slipped into a coma and was hooked up to a ventilator to keep him breathing.

The next day, while his family and doctors feared the worst, Dr. McIver woke up. He learned that he'd had a massive heart attack, caused by blockage in his coronary artery feeding the

> " You should never ignore symptoms when it involves pain in the chest. And don't diagnose yourself. I'm a doctor and I didn't get it right. "

front of his heart — an artery that many doctors refer to as the "widow-maker."

Dr. McIver considers himself lucky to have been at a hospital when the plaques in his artery ruptured, triggering the heart attack. "I'm a living testament to the fact that modern technology really does save lives, and that good medical care matters," he says. "The reason I lived was because of prompt CPR, immediate therapy to restore the blood supply with a stent and incredibly skilled intensive care."

His physical recovery progressed smoothly, but recovering psychologically took a little longer. "It was emotionally trying," he says. "I learned that physical disease has psychological consequences."

One of his ongoing challenges has been balancing work with a healthy lifestyle. "I continue to struggle with exercise," he says. "I love cycling and skiing, and so forth, but to go and walk on the treadmill or cycle on the stationary bike drives me crazy — I hate it with a passion. I have to force myself to do those things."

He understands how difficult it can be to adopt healthier habits. But he urges his patients with diabetes to try to manage the disease with lifestyle changes rather than drugs. The effort can make a dramatic difference in slowing down the progression of diabetes — and reducing the risk of heart disease, which is higher among people with diabetes.

CHAPTER 16

HEART FAILURE

Heart failure sounds scary, and to be sure, it's a serious problem. But it doesn't mean that your heart has totally stopped working. Rather, it means your heart is not doing its job as well as it should. The heart muscle has become too weak or too stiff to pump enough blood to meet your body's needs.

Heart failure often develops after other conditions, such as heart attack or arrhythmias, have damaged the heart. The main pumping chambers — the ventricles — become weakened and stretched (dilated), unable to pump blood with much force. Or the ventricles become stiff and don't fill with enough blood between heartbeats, causing blood to back up into the lungs, liver, abdomen, or legs and feet (congestion). Heart failure also may occur because your heart simply can't pump enough blood to meet the demand.

> " I exercise on an elliptical machine. The nurses were worried about me doing so much with my artificial heart pump, but my doctors said it was fine. It bothers me that some people won't take care of themselves, even when they've been given a second chance at life. "

Jacqueline

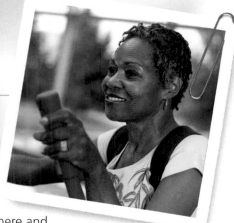

Diagnosis: Dilated cardiomyopathy

Heart story: Jacqueline, 56, was always on the run. Work, being a mom, wife and grandmother, she loved it all. She also had a passion for running. But a few years ago, she found herself slowing down. "It wasn't as easy to get out there and run," she says. "I really had to force myself. I attributed it to working too much." Over the next year she noticed that she had increasing shortness of breath. She was diagnosed with a rare disease called sarcoidosis that damaged her heart, leading to severe heart failure. When medications were no longer effective, doctors told her she needed a heart transplant or a heart pump (left ventricular assist device) if she was to survive.

Outcome: While waiting for a transplant, Jacqueline received a left ventricular assist device. She made a new commitment to exercise and feels great. She goes to the gym four or five days a week. She's not quite as fast as she used to be, but it doesn't bother her. "You can't dwell on, 'Oh, I'm locked down with this.' Dwell on the fact that you've got life, and you'll see your life improve day by day. You've got to think about the possibilities, not the limitations."

Dilated cardiomyopathy

In this common form of cardiomyopathy, weakened heart muscle reduces the ability of the heart to pump blood with force. The left ventricle enlarges (dilates) to compensate for its reduced ability to pump blood to the body.

Left ventricle

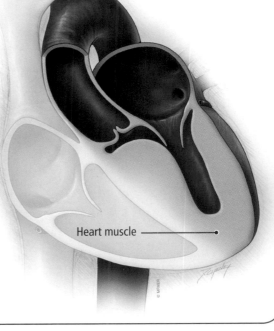

Hypertrophic cardiomyopathy

With this condition, abnormally thickened (hypertrophied) muscle interferes with the heart's ability to fill the left ventricle with blood and may obstruct the flow of blood leaving the heart.

Heart muscle

Causes

A variety of medical conditions can reduce your heart's ability to pump blood effectively. Heart failure can involve the left side, right side or both sides of your heart. Causes include:

+ **Coronary artery disease.** The No. 1 form of heart disease is also the most common cause of heart failure.

+ **Diabetes.** Persistently high levels of blood sugar can damage the heart muscle.

+ **High blood pressure.** Your heart works harder when it's under high pressure.

+ **Faulty heart valves.** A defective valve forces your heart to work harder to keep blood flowing as it should.

+ **Birth defects of the heart.** Congenital abnormalities affect heart function.

+ **Abnormal heart rhythms (arrhythmias).** Fast heartbeats can weaken heart muscle; slow heartbeats may prevent enough blood getting to the body.

+ **Myocarditis.** Inflammation of the heart muscle, usually caused by a virus, can affect heart function.

+ **Cardiomyopathy.** This heart muscle disease can lead to heart failure. Common types include:

  » **Dilated cardiomyopathy —** When the heart muscle becomes weak and pumps less forcefully, the heart enlarges (dilates) to compensate. Often, a cause isn't known, but it can run in families or be caused by factors such as alcohol use or chemotherapy.

  » **Hypertrophic cardiomyopathy** — The heart muscle becomes abnormally thick and stiff, interfering with its ability to pump blood. This condition is usually inherited.

  » **Restrictive cardiomyopathy** — The heart muscle becomes rigid, so the heart can't properly expand and fill with blood. It may occur with no apparent cause, or from disease such as amyloidosis, when abnormal deposits build up in the heart.

Symptoms

Heart failure can be ongoing (chronic) or start suddenly, with new or recurrent symptoms (acute). Symptoms may include:

- Shortness of breath when you exert yourself or when you're lying down
- Fatigue and weakness
- Swelling in your legs, ankles and feet
- Rapid or irregular heartbeat
- Reduced ability to exercise
- Persistent cough or wheezing with white or pink phlegm
- Swelling of your abdomen
- Sudden weight gain
- Lack of appetite and nausea
- Difficulty concentrating or decreased alertness

What's 'congestive' about heart failure?

A damaged or weakened heart can cause what is commonly called congestive heart failure (see Chapter 14). As blood flowing out of the heart and through the arteries slows down, blood flowing into the heart through the veins backs up, causing fluid to collect in or congest body tissue. If heart failure affects the left side of your

Broken heart syndrome

A woman receives terrible news that her husband has died of a heart attack. Soon she's also experiencing what seems to be a heart attack. A condition called "broken heart" syndrome (stress cardiomyopathy) may occur in the wake of highly stressful emotional or physical situations, such as traumas or accidents. Symptoms often mimic a heart attack, but in this case chest pain doesn't stem from coronary blockage. Instead, part of the heart — typically the left ventricle — is temporarily weakened. Most people who have broken heart syndrome make a full recovery after a short hospital stay.

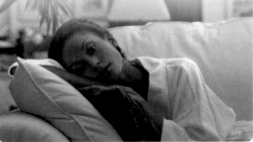

heart, the left ventricle acts more like a dam than a pump, and blood backs up in your lungs, leading to shortness of breath and fatigue.

In right-sided heart failure, pressure causes fluid to collect in your abdomen, legs and feet. This causes swelling (edema), most often in your legs and ankles. Heart failure also stimulates the kidneys to retain more sodium and water in your system, another cause of swelling. Abdominal symptoms might include nausea, pain, loss of appetite and bloating.

Diagnosis and treatment

Your doctor can diagnose heart failure based on your medical history, a general physical exam and a variety of test results. No single test can determine whether you have heart failure.

Common tests to diagnose heart failure include chest X-ray, electrocardiogram, echocardiogram and blood tests, such as the B-type natriuretic peptide (BNP) test. The level of the BNP hormone increases in your bloodstream as heart failure develops.

A common measure of your heart's pumping function is known as your "ejection fraction." (See Chapter 14.) This is a measure, expressed as a percentage, of how much blood leaves your heart's main pumping chamber, the left ventricle, each time it contracts. A normal ejection fraction is 50 to 70 percent. A lower percentage is a sign that your heart muscle is weak. However, heart failure can also occur even if your ejection fraction is in the normal range. This may happen if your heart muscle becomes stiff from conditions such as high blood pressure.

Cases of heart failure range in severity. Doctors sometimes can correct the underlying problem, but for most people, heart failure is a condition requiring lifelong management. A combination of medications are used to improve your symptoms and heart function and help you live longer. Lifestyle changes, such as to diet and exercise, are important, as well.

Some people with heart failure may benefit from implantable heart devices. These devices include implantable cardioverter-defibrillators (ICDs) to prevent sudden cardiac death, special pacemakers to coordinate the electrical system of the heart (biventricular pacemakers), or mechanical heart pumps (left ventricular assist devices, or LVADs) to improve blood flow.

A Healthy Heart Plan
for heart failure

If you have heart failure, these steps
can help you stay with your plan.

1 **Treat salt as the enemy.** Whatever
pleasure they bring, salty foods
just aren't worth it. Sodium aggravates
the symptoms of heart failure because it
draws more fluid into your bloodstream,
increasing the total volume of blood in
your system and making your already
weakened heart work even harder.

Educate yourself about the ways salt
can creep into your diet. You can often
reduce the amount of salt you use
simply by eating more fresh vegetables
and fruits. Avoid high-sodium foods,
such as many canned or baked goods,
processed meats and cheese. Also, be
cautious about using salt substitutes.
Some of these products may be high in
potassium, and your doctor might not
recommend them.

2 **Weigh yourself each morning
before breakfast.** Weight gain
can signal the start of congestion in
your lungs, abdomen or legs. Learn to
recognize symptoms that indicate heart
failure is getting worse, including:

- Sudden weight gain of 3 or more pounds over a day or two
- Increased swelling, shortness of breath or fatigue
- Increased frequency or severity of chest pain
- Inability to lie flat at night due to shortness of breath or cough

3 **Watch how much you drink.** With heart failure, too much fluid makes your heart work too hard. If you can imagine your heart as a pump, you need just enough fluid in your body to keep the pump "primed" but not so much as to flood the system. So, if your doctor prescribes a certain amount of fluid to drink every day, try not to exceed that limit. At the same time, don't risk dehydration. If you still feel thirsty, try this:

- Rinse your mouth with water often
- Brush your teeth more often
- Suck on sugar-free hard candy or frozen grapes or lemon bits
- Keep your lips moist with lip balm

4 **Exercise safely.** If you're tired or short of breath, you might not feel like bicycling or walking. But even people with heart failure and shortness

Specialist focus:

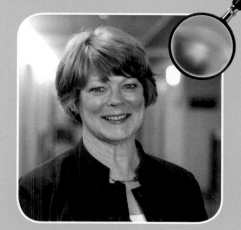

Cindy R. Truex, R.N., specializes in educating and caring for heart failure patients at Mayo Clinic.

Most people are really scared when they hear the term *heart failure*. It's better to think of this diagnosis as a change of heart function rather than failure. It's also important for you to be an actively involved member of your treatment team in order to have the best response to therapy. Sometimes you might temporarily feel worse before you feel better. But if your heart improves, it's all worth it.

of breath can benefit from regular activity — provided it's tailored to your condition. Ask your doctor what's right for you.

5 **Pace yourself.** Maintain about the same level of daily activity, and rest following difficult tasks. Try scoring activities from 1 (light) to 5 (hard). Never group 4s and 5s close together. Space them throughout the week.

After morning chores, relax and avoid something else that's physically taxing until late afternoon. Whenever you're short of breath or tired from exercise, take a break. Even with severe heart failure, you can usually remain active, as long as you are realistic in planning your schedule.

6 **Watch your levels of potassium.** Some heart failure medications can affect your body's level of potassium, a mineral important for your heart health. Low potassium levels can cause dangerous heart rhythm problems. Talk to your doctor about any changes in your diet that might be needed because of the medications you're on.

7 **Get checked for sleep disorders.** As many as half of people with heart failure have sleep apnea. Despite this connection, sleep disorders often go undiagnosed in people with heart failure. One reason is that the symptoms of sleep apnea and heart failure often overlap, disguising the cause.

In addition, many people who have both conditions don't feel sleepy during the day, so they're not aware that they have a sleep disorder. Ask your doctor about the need to screen for conditions such as sleep apnea.

8 **Ask about family screening.** Some types of cardiomyopathy may be inherited. Your doctor may recommend screening for family members, including a physical exam, electrocardiogram, echocardiogram, genetic screening and

Understand your medications

If you're like most people with heart failure, you could be taking nine to 12 pills a day. Understand the purpose of each medication and have a system in place for taking the drugs as prescribed. Plan ahead for refills. You may feel temporarily worse as your body adjusts to the drugs, but don't stop taking them without medical advice. Sometimes you may need a change of dose or just a little more time to get used to a drug. Many of these medications can improve your heart and help you live longer.

Drug type	Action
Vasodilators	Relax your blood vessels and reduce your heart's workload, decreasing the chance of heart enlargement. Examples include angiotensin-converting enzyme (ACE) inhibitors and angiotensin receptor blockers (ARBs).
Beta blockers	Ease the heart's workload and risk of some abnormal heart rhythms, and may improve heart function.
Aldosterone antagonists	May reverse scarring of the heart muscle and help remove fluid.
Digoxin	Improves heart muscle contraction strength and tends to slow the heartbeat.
Diuretics (water pills)	Make you urinate more frequently and keep fluid from collecting in the body.

genetic counseling. Early treatment can prevent heart failure and sudden death.

9 **Find out if you need an ICD.** Some people with heart failure or cardiomyopathy will have a higher risk of dangerous heart rhythms. An ICD monitors your heart rhythms and can treat dangerous, life-threatening heart rhythms with pacing or by delivering an electrical shock.

- -

➜ **Additional resources:**

Mayo Clinic
www.mayoclinic.com

National Heart, Lung, and Blood Institute
www.nhlbi.nih.gov

Heart Failure Society of America
www.hfsa.org

Hypertrophic Cardiomyopathy Association
www.4hcm.org

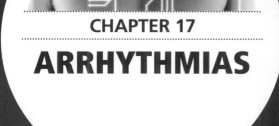

CHAPTER 17

ARRHYTHMIAS

Many people experience an occasional fluttering of their heart, especially during stressful times, or when exercising. But when does the occasional fluttering become a concern? Or what does it mean when your doctor tells you that there may be a problem with your heart's rhythm that you didn't know anything about?

If you sometimes feel like your heart is racing or skipping a beat for a short time, it's probably not cause for alarm. But, if an abnormal heartbeat persists, it could signal that something is amiss in the pathways through which your heart's electrical signal travels. Heart rhythm problems are called arrhythmias. Sometimes, you may have no symptoms of an arrhythmia and may be surprised to learn you have one.

> " I can dance all night long now. Before, I was so tired that I had to sit down after every song. "

Francisco

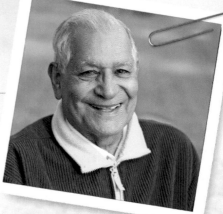

Diagnosis: Atrial fibrillation

Event: Francisco loves to move. In his 40 years as a physical education teacher, he showed countless children the importance of physical activity. And it's not just sports that are his passion. Francisco, a huge music fan, loves to dance. But when Francisco turned 75 he began noticing a problem with his heart rhythm. "It felt like my heart was beating too hard," he explains. "And when I bent over, I felt light-headed." Dancing became more difficult. When he and his wife of 52 years went dancing, he had to frequently sit down and rest. Francisco's primary care doctor diagnosed him with atrial fibrillation, a common heart problem that causes your heart to beat irregularly or too quickly. Although Francisco's symptoms were severe, he was able to be treated effectively with medications to slow his heart rate and a blood thinner to prevent strokes.

Outcome: Francisco is dancing again. In fact, he attended a 15th birthday party for one of his granddaughters and amazed the guests with his fancy footwork. "He was dancing with all of my daughter's friends. I think he tired them out," says Francisco's daughter, Carmen. Francisco says he's glad to get back to living life to the fullest. Don't let heart problems discourage you, he says. Listen to your doctor, and take care of the problem. "You have to live every single minute of your life," he says.

Arrhythmias are often harmless. You may need nothing more than reassurance from your doctor that the condition isn't caused by anything serious. If treatment is required, medications are often effective. Sometimes you may need a device, such as a pacemaker or defibrillator, or an invasive procedure to correct the heart rhythm.

Causes

Arrhythmias are caused by abnormalities along the pathway that your heart's electrical signals travel to make your heart beat.

These abnormalities can be caused by underlying heart disease, such as a heart attack or cardiomyopathy, which affects the structure of your heart or causes scarring in heart muscle tissue. Sometimes arrhythmias can be hereditary, without any abnormalities in the heart's structure.

Other health problems, such as high blood pressure, diabetes, sleep apnea or other sleep disorders, or a thyroid disorder can disturb the heart's rhythm. Arrhythmias can also be brought on by medications, smoking,

alcohol, illegal drugs, and the use of stimulants such as dietary supplements, caffeine and energy drinks.

Doctors classify arrhythmias not only by where they originate in the heart but also by the speed of heart rate they cause:

+ **Tachycardia.** This refers to a fast heartbeat — a resting heart rate greater than 100 beats a minute.

+ **Bradycardia.** This refers to a slow heartbeat — a resting heart rate less than 60 beats a minute.

Tachycardias can occur in the upper or lower chambers of your heart. Some tachycardias in the upper chambers of your heart (atria) can be nothing more than a nuisance that's uncomfortable.

Atrial fibrillation or atrial flutter — a form of tachycardia — can be more serious. These arrhythmias can cause blood clots to form, increasing your risk for heart attack or stroke.

Tachycardias in the lower chambers of your heart (ventricles) are often very dangerous. During persistent

Normal heartbeat

The process begins when a tiny cluster of cells at the sinus node (SA) sends out an electrical signal. The signal travels through the atria to the atrioventricular (AV) node and then passes into the ventricles, causing them to contract and pump out blood.

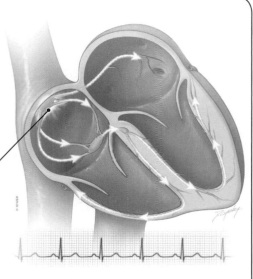

Sinus
node

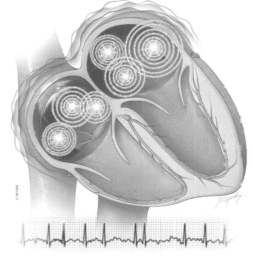

Atrial fibrillation

Electrical signals fire from multiple locations in the atria, causing the atria to beat chaotically, irregularly and out of coordination with the two lower chambers (ventricles) of the heart. The ventricles respond to these chaotic signals by beating faster.

Ventricular fibrillation

Rapid, erratic electrical impulses occur in the ventricles, causing them to quiver uselessly instead of pumping blood. Within a few seconds, a person with ventricular fibrillation will collapse, stop breathing and lose his or her pulse. The condition is fatal unless treated immediately with CPR and defibrillation.

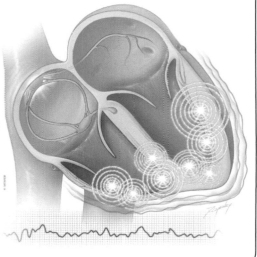

Ventricular fibrillation — a deadly arrhythmia

In ventricular fibrillation, rapid, chaotic electrical impulses cause your ventricles to quiver uselessly instead of pumping blood. Without an effective heartbeat, your blood pressure plummets, cutting off blood supply to your vital organs — including your brain. Most people lose consciousness within seconds and require immediate medical assistance, including cardiopulmonary resuscitation (CPR). Without CPR or defibrillation, death results in minutes. Most cases of ventricular fibrillation are linked to some form of heart disease. Ventricular fibrillation is frequently triggered by a heart attack.

ventricular tachycardia, the heart cannot pump enough blood to your body, resulting in fainting, organ damage and cardiac arrest. Ventricular tachycardia can deteriorate into a deadly rhythm called ventricular fibrillation.

Bradycardias can be caused by a problem with the sinus node, your heart's natural pacemaker that produces the signals that cause your heart to beat (sick sinus syndrome). They can also be caused by blockage of the pathway between the upper and lower chambers of your heart (atrioventricular block). If the bradycardia causes your heart to beat so slowly that the rest of your body doesn't receive enough blood, you may faint, fatigue easily or develop other heart problems, such as heart failure.

Symptoms

Arrhythmias may not cause any signs or symptoms. In fact, your doctor might detect an arrhythmia during a routine examination before you notice it.

Arrhythmia signs and symptoms may include:

✔ Fluttering in the chest
✔ Racing heartbeat
✔ Slow heartbeat
✔ Skipped heartbeats
✔ Chest pain
✔ Shortness of breath
✔ Difficulty performing exercise
✔ Lightheadedness
✔ Dizziness
✔ Fainting (syncope) or near fainting

Complishcations

+ **Stroke.** During atrial fibrillation, the upper chambers of your heart (atria) aren't beating effectively and blood clots may form, especially in older people and those who have other heart problems. If a clot breaks loose, it can travel to and obstruct a brain artery, causing a stroke. For people who have atrial fibrillation, blood-thinning medications are often recommended to reduce the risk of stroke.

+ **Heart failure.** This can result if your heart is pumping ineffectively for a prolonged period due to a bradycardia or tachycardia, such as atrial fibrillation. Sometimes, controlling the rate of an arrhythmia that's causing heart failure can improve your heart's function.

Diagnosis and treatment

Your doctor will likely want to check the electrical activity of your heart using an electrocardiogram (ECG or EKG), a noninvasive test that measures the impulses that make your heart beat. The test uses electrodes connected to a monitor or printer. An

Sudden cardiac death in athletes and young people

You've probably heard reports of young athletes who have dropped dead because of an undiagnosed heart problem. Typically, such an event — sudden cardiac death — is due to an unrecognized heart condition. The most common cause of sudden cardiac death in athletes and people under 30 is hypertrophic cardiomyopathy (described on page 159), an inherited muscle disorder. Other inherited conditions, such as long QT syndrome, Brugada syndrome and arrhythmogenic right ventricular cardiomyopathy (ARVC) may also be responsible.

Many times, these deaths occur with no warning, but there are two red flags to watch for: Unexplained fainting and a family history of sudden cardiac death. Symptoms such as shortness of breath or chest pain with exercise may be a sign of increased risk, but are uncommon and more often due to other health problems, such as asthma.

electrocardiogram can help your doctor figure out what type of arrhythmia you have. Other types of electrocardiograms, such as holter monitoring and event recording, can help in instances when the arrhythmias only occur occasionally.

Your doctor may also order imaging tests of your heart, such as an echo-cardiogram, computerized tomography (CT), magnetic resonance imaging (MRI) or cardiac catheterization. These tests give your doctor information about your heart's size, structure and motion.

Treatment for an arrhythmia often isn't necessary unless the arrhythmia is causing significant symptoms or is putting you at risk of a more serious arrhythmia or complication. Your doctor will recommend healthy lifestyle changes no matter what your arrhythmia.

Ablation: An arrhythmia treatment

Cardiac ablation is a procedure that can correct heart rhythm problems. Ablation typically uses catheters — long, flexible tubes inserted through a vein in your groin and threaded to your heart — to correct structural problems in your heart that cause an arrhythmia. Occasionally, cardiac ablation is done through open-heart surgery, usually at the time of another procedure, such as cardiac valve surgery.

Cardiac ablation works by scarring or destroying the tissue in your heart that triggers an abnormal heart rhythm. In some cases, ablation prevents abnormal electrical signals from traveling through your heart, thus stopping the arrhythmia. Ablation isn't usually a first treatment option, but it is a treatment option for people who:

+ Have unsuccessfully tried medications to treat arrhythmias
+ Have had serious side effects from medications to treat arrhythmias
+ Have certain types of arrhythmias that respond well to ablation, such as Wolff-Parkinson-White syndrome
+ Have a high risk of complications from arrhythmias, such as sudden cardiac arrest

Your doctor may prescribe medications to speed up or slow down your heart rate, if necessary. If you have atrial fibrillation, your doctor may recommend electrical cardioversion, a procedure in which your heart is shocked into a normal rhythm while you're under sedation. If your arrhythmia is serious, you may need medication, ablation or surgery.

Adapting the Healthy Heart Plan to arrhythmias

Many arrhythmias can be blamed on underlying heart disease, so following the components of the Healthy Heart Plan is essential to treating your arrhythmia. To tailor the plan to your condition, you should also:

1 **Get your doctor's OK before exercising.** Exercise is an important part of the Mayo Clinic Healthy Heart Plan, but if you have an arrhythmia, it's wise to check with your doctor before starting regular exercise. If you have atrial fibrillation, it's important to make sure your heart doesn't race too fast from exercise. Your heart rate may speed up quickly as soon as you exert yourself.

2 **Ask your doctor about blood-thinning medications.** Some people who have an arrhythmia — especially atrial fibrillation — have a risk of developing blood clots that can cause a stroke. Talk to your doctor about your blood-clotting risks, and if you need blood-thinning medication. If you need medication, take it exactly as prescribed and let other health care providers know you're taking a blood thinner.

3 **Cut back on caffeine and alcohol.** Caffeine can cause your heart to beat faster and may contribute to the development of more-serious arrhythmias. Drinking too much alcohol can affect the electrical impulses in your heart or increase the chance of developing both short-term and chronic arrhythmias. Chronic alcohol abuse may cause your heart to beat less effectively and can weaken the heart muscle (alcoholic cardiomyopathy).

Specialist focus:

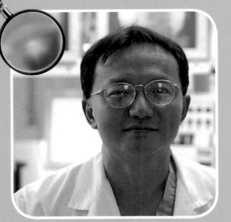

Win-Kuang Shen, M.D., is an expert on arrhythmias at Mayo Clinic.

Different arrhythmias can cause similar symptoms, so connecting the symptoms to a precise rhythm disturbance is important. Some people pay little attention to occasional palpitations, even though they represent a life-threatening condition. Other people think that having occasional palpitations means they'll keel over tomorrow from a sudden cardiac event — even though the palpitations are harmless. Getting a precise diagnosis allows you to understand your condition much better.

4 **Quit using tobacco products.**
Not only can the chemicals in tobacco damage your arteries, but the nicotine in cigarettes and chewing tobacco can also speed up your heart rate, worsening an arrhythmia. Talk to your doctor about ways to quit smoking or chewing tobacco if you're concerned about your ability to stop.

5 **Ask your doctor if you need an implanted medical device.**
Depending on what type of arrhythmia you have, you may benefit from having a pacemaker or implantable cardio-verter-defibrillator (ICD) implanted in your chest.

A pacemaker can help people with slow heart rates. If a pacemaker detects a heart rate that's too slow or no heart-beat at all, it emits electrical impulses that stimulate your heart to speed up or begin beating again.

An ICD can help if you're at risk of developing a dangerously fast heartbeat, or if your heart slows or stops. The ICD continuously monitors your heart rhythm. If it detects a rhythm that's too slow, it paces the heart as a pacemaker would. If it detects a fast heartbeat, it sends out low- or high-energy shocks to reset the heart to a normal rhythm.

Both devices require minimally invasive surgery to implant and may be life-saving if you're a good candidate for the device.

6 **Find ways to reduce the amount of stress in your life.** Your body produces a surge of hormones when you're in a stressful situation. These hormones temporarily increase your blood pressure by causing your heart to beat faster and your blood vessels to narrow, which can put added stress on your heart if you have an arrhythmia. Take a few moments each day to relax, and try to figure out what your stressors are in order to better deal with them or avoid them.

7 **Be cautious with over-the-counter medications and supplements.** Stimulant medications, such as over-the-counter cold medicines, can speed up your heart rate. Check with your doctor before taking any over-the-counter medications or supplements as they could worsen your arrhythmia or interact with other medications you're taking.

→ **Additional resources:**

Mayo Clinic
www.mayoclinic.com

Heart Rhythm Society
www.hrsonline.org

National Heart, Lung, and Blood Institute
www.nhlbi.nih.gov

CHAPTER 18

HEART VALVE DISORDERS

Heart valve disorders can be a stealthy problem. They often go undetected for years, without causing symptoms. These disorders typically show up in older adults, and will likely become more common as the general population ages.

Four valves keep blood flowing through the four chambers of the heart (for more, see Chapter 14). The valves consist of strong, thin flaps of tissue, called leaflets, which open and close with each heartbeat. When the pressure of blood pushes against the leaflets, they swing open like one-way gates and blood passes through. When the pressure lessens, the leaflets close, preventing blood from moving backward. The valves allow blood to flow in only one direction through the heart.

" My doctors gave me strict rules to live by, and I realized that if I wanted to live, I should follow those rules. I did, and I'm here today, thanks to God. I'm living better than I've ever lived in my life. "

Sidney

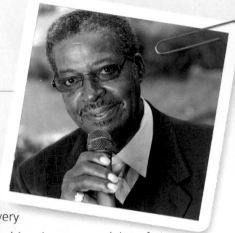

Diagnosis: Tricuspid valve regurgitation

Event: Sidney was an active outdoor enthusiast. He loved to hunt and fish. When he wasn't outside, he enjoyed singing in his church choir. He developed symptoms that prompted a heart valve replacement, and made a full recovery from the procedure. But a few years later, his primary complaint of coughing returned. He had developed leakage (regurgitation) of the tricuspid valve, causing severe heart failure. The condition caused his kidneys and liver to fail. His only option was a high-risk valve surgery or going into hospice care.

Outcome: Today Sidney feels great. Singing is no longer a problem, and he's enjoying spending time outdoors. For him, he says the difference was having faith in God, his doctors' advice and a new attitude. "You've got to have faith. You can't just lay there and fade away," Sidney says. "I had to change my lifestyle and my eating habits. I joined the health club and go at least three times a week. Salt was one of the biggest problems for me. I completely cut out salt. We think we need salt for taste, but we don't. I don't eat a lot of fried foods. We barbecue, bake and broil a lot. I'm an outdoorsman, and I catch a lot of fish. There's a way to cook fish without salt that tastes good."

In heart valve disorders, one of the heart valves fails to open or close properly. This disrupts the efficient flow of blood through the heart. Two major problems can happen to the valves: narrowing of the valve opening (stenosis) and leakage of blood back through the valve opening (regurgitation).

Stenosis. When a valve becomes narrowed, it can't open fully. This smaller opening slows or blocks blood flow, and your heart has to work harder to pump an adequate amount of blood to your body.

Regurgitation. When a valve doesn't close tightly, some blood leaks backward instead of flowing forward through the heart or into an artery. This inefficient blood flow can cause your heart to work harder.

Eventually, a heart valve disorder may require surgery to either repair or replace the faulty valve.

Some of the most common types of heart valve disorders include:

- **Aortic stenosis.** This occurs when the heart's aortic valve narrows.

The narrowing prevents the valve from opening fully, which obstructs blood flow from your heart into your aorta and onward to the rest of your body.

- **Mitral stenosis.** This happens when the heart's mitral valve narrows. The abnormal valve doesn't open properly, blocking blood flow coming into your left ventricle, the main pumping chamber of your heart.

- **Aortic regurgitation.** This occurs when your heart's aortic valve doesn't close tightly. This allows some of the blood that was just pumped out of your heart's main pumping chamber (left ventricle) to leak back into it.

- **Mitral regurgitation.** This happens when your heart's mitral valve doesn't close tightly, which allows blood to flow backward in your heart.

Causes

Heart valves may not work properly for a variety of reasons, which many times will cause the valve to weaken, stiffen or deteriorate over time. Here is a list of common causes:

Mitral valve prolapse

With this disorder, the leaflets of the mitral valve bulge (prolapse) into the left atrium like a parachute during the heart's contraction. Sometimes mitral valve prolapse causes blood to leak back into the atrium from the ventricle (see bold arrows on the image). This is called mitral valve regurgitation. The inset image shows a ruptured mitral valve chord — a complication of mitral prolapse that can cause regurgitation.

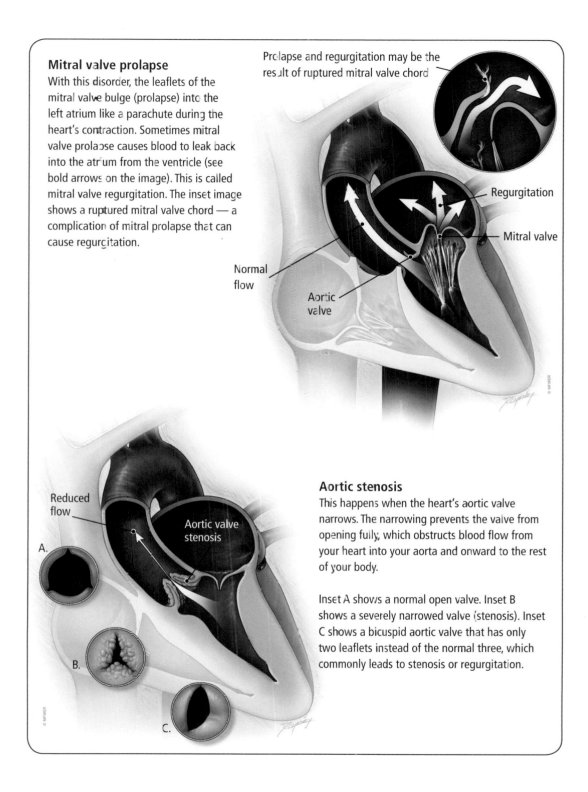

Prolapse and regurgitation may be the result of ruptured mitral valve chord

Regurgitation

Mitral valve

Normal flow

Aortic valve

Reduced flow

Aortic valve stenosis

A.

B.

C.

Aortic stenosis

This happens when the heart's aortic valve narrows. The narrowing prevents the valve from opening fully, which obstructs blood flow from your heart into your aorta and onward to the rest of your body.

Inset A shows a normal open valve. Inset B shows a severely narrowed valve (stenosis). Inset C shows a bicuspid aortic valve that has only two leaflets instead of the normal three, which commonly leads to stenosis or regurgitation.

Calcium buildup. Calcium is an abundant mineral in your body that's carried in your bloodstream. As you age, deposits of calcium may accumulate on your aortic valve. The deposits stiffen and thicken the valve leaflets, narrowing the valve opening and limiting the volume of blood flow. Many of the risk factors for developing calcium deposits are the same as for developing atherosclerosis (for more, see page 138) — they include diabetes, high blood pressure, smoking and high cholesterol.

Wear and tear. Your heart valves open and shut tens of thousands of times a day, every day of your life. With advanced age, the wear and tear of all this activity may cause a valve to weaken or deteriorate, leading to regurgitation.

Rheumatic fever. In developing countries, the major cause of heart valve disease is rheumatic fever, which is a complication of strep throat infection. The disease can leave lasting damage or scarring of the heart valves. While rheumatic fever is rare in the United States, some older people may have had it as children.

When valve disorders become emergencies

Most heart valve disorders cause no or mild symptoms over many years. But some valve problems can develop suddenly and require immediate medical attention. Warning signs include:

+ Severe or sudden shortness of breath
+ Rapid breathing or pulse
+ Fainting
+ Altered mental state
+ Severe chest pain

Birth defects. Some people are born with a heart valve defect, such as an aortic valve that has only two leaflets instead of the normal three (bicuspid aortic valve). In a condition called mitral valve prolapse, the mitral valve's leaflets don't meet together in the middle of the valve as they should, causing the valve to leak.

Infections. An infection inside the heart — known as infective endocarditis — can cause or worsen heart valve disease.

Other causes. A prior heart attack, untreated high blood pressure, certain medications, previous radiation treatment or inflammatory conditions such as lupus also may be responsible for heart valve problems.

Symptoms

Most heart valve disorders develop very slowly. You may have no symptoms for decades. Signs and symptoms include:

- Fatigue, especially during times of increased activity
- Shortness of breath, especially with exertion or when lying down
- Abnormal sounds heard during a heartbeat (heart murmur)
- Feeling faint or fainting
- Rapid, fluttering heartbeat (palpitations)
- Irregular heartbeat
- Chest pain, discomfort or tightness
- Swollen ankles and feet
- Coughing

Complications

Heart failure. A narrowed valve can reduce the flow of blood through your heart or cause pressure to build up in your lungs, putting additional strain on the heart. Your heart may become too weak to pump enough blood to meet your body's needs.

Abnormal heart rhythm (arrhythmia). Damage to muscle tissue in the heart interferes with the electrical impulses that coordinate your heartbeats. This may cause abnormal heart rhythms — the heart beats too fast, too slow or irregularly.

Chest pain (angina). Reduced blood flow to your heart often causes chest pain. This is a common symptom of severe aortic stenosis, when not enough blood is pumped into your main artery, the aorta. The discomfort is typically triggered by physical or emotional stress and goes away soon after stopping the stressful activity.

Infection (endocarditis). A diseased or damaged valve is more prone to infection than is a healthy valve.

Lung problems. Some valve disorders can cause blood and fluid to back up in your lungs (congestion) or trigger high blood pressure in your lungs (pulmonary hypertension).

Diagnosis and treatment

For many people, a heart murmur is the first sign of a heart valve disorder. An important test in diagnosing heart valve disease is an echocardiogram, which is an ultrasound of your heart. Other tests include an electrocardiogram, chest X-ray, stress test, cardiac magnetic resonance imaging (MRI) and cardiac catheterization. For more information on these tests, see Chapter 21.

The main treatment for a heart valve disorder is surgery to repair or replace the valve. New techniques make it possible to fix some valves without open-heart surgery. But you might not need surgery right away — or ever.

If you have mild to moderate valve stenosis or regurgitation and no symptoms, you'll have regular checkups to monitor the valve. If your condition gets worse — even if you don't have symptoms — your doctor might recommend repairing or replacing the valve. Mitral and tricuspid valves often can be repaired, but aortic and pulmonary valves usually require replacement.

Medications can't cure a heart valve disorder, but they do have a role in treatment. Your doctor might prescribe drugs that help ease symptoms, control high blood pressure, lower cholesterol, reduce fluid buildup or prevent blood clots, as needed.

Heart murmurs

A common diagnosis for children and adults is a heart murmur. Heart murmurs are abnormal sounds during your heartbeat cycle — such as whooshing or swishing — made by turbulent blood in or near your heart. A heart murmur may be the first sign your doctor detects when diagnosing a heart valve problem. A heart murmur could also be a sign of other heart problems, such as a congenital defect.

While most heart murmurs are harmless, a murmur could signal there's a problem in the structure of your heart, such as a leaking or hardened valve, or abnormal blood flow. If you're diagnosed with a heart murmur, your doctor may order more tests to check the cause of the murmur.

An echocardiogram can show how severe a valve problem is and, if it's getting worse, how fast it's progressing. The test can also indicate how well your heart is working. Actively observing the stability or progression of a heart valve condition is important so that you can receive the right treatment at the right time.

If you aren't experiencing any symptoms, how often you'll need checkups depends on the severity of your condition. If your valve is leaking badly, for example, you might need to have an echocardiogram every six to 12 months. That's because if you wait too long before having surgery, your heart might become damaged beyond repair or become so weakened that surgery wouldn't help to correct it.

It's also important to keep an eye out for the onset of heart valve symptoms. If you have aortic stenosis, for example, symptoms develop when the narrowing becomes severe and you'll need surgery to repair or replace the valve. Close monitoring is important because, left untreated, the heart-weakening effects of aortic stenosis can lead to heart failure.

Specialist focus:

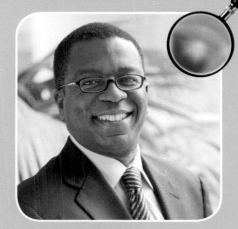

Vuyisile T. Nkomo, M.D., is an expert in valvular heart disease at Mayo Clinic.

A lot of people think that fatigue and shortness of breath are just a part of getting old, but these are also common symptoms of a heart valve disorder. If you notice that other people in your age group are able to be more active than you are without becoming winded or fatigued, then you should schedule a visit with your doctor and be checked for heart valve disease.

A Healthy Heart Plan for heart valve disorders

Add these steps into your Healthy Heart Plan if you have a heart valve disorder.

1 **See your doctor if you develop symptoms.** Because heart valve disorders often don't cause symptoms until late in the disease, their presence may signal a change and the need for valve replacement. Watch for new symptoms that could indicate a turn for the worse, such as:

- ✔ Chest pain
- ✔ Dizziness
- ✔ Fatigue and weakness
- ✔ Shortness of breath
- ✔ Swelling
- ✔ Rapid or irregular heartbeat
- ✔ Reduced ability to exercise

You might ask family or friends to keep an eye out as well. It's not uncommon for people with heart valve disorders to not recognize symptoms or to start limiting their activity — either consciously or unconsciously — as the symptoms progress, which can mask the seriousness of the disease.

2 **Exercise safely.** Understand your exercise limitations, if any. Some people with valve disease can run marathons, while others need to stick with low-intensity activities, such as walking, bowling or golf. To help determine your specific limits, your doctor might do exercise testing to check blood pressure and other signs and symptoms while you're exerting yourself at a particular intensity level. Bottom line: Learn how the disease specifically affects you and recognize the symptoms that signal trouble. Also, start slowly with any new physical activity, drink plenty of water when exercising, and stop your activity immediately if you develop symptoms such as shortness of breath or lightheadedness.

3 **Ask if you need antibiotics before having dental work.** In the past, people with heart valve disorders were advised to take antibiotics before dental procedures in order to help prevent infections (endocarditis) developing in the heart. According to new guidelines, most people with heart valve disease don't need to take this precaution. However, the guidelines still apply to people who are at especially high risk of possible problems from an infection.

Remember that good dental hygiene and regular dental care are important for anyone with heart disease.

④ Check if your immediate family may need to be screened. If you learn that your heart valve disorder has a genetic or hereditary component, ask your doctor if family members should be screened to see if they also have the disorder. For example, many heart specialists recommend that first-degree relatives — parents, siblings, children — of people with bicuspid aortic valve (BAV) disease be screened with echocardiography, since BAV tends to run in families.

⑤ Stay in shape for a possible surgery. If you have a heart valve disorder, you may need surgery at some point. Over time — often many years — these disorders may get worse, and to prevent lasting damage to your heart, the valve has to be replaced or repaired. For most people, this will mean open-heart surgery. The healthier you are going into it, the better your chances of doing well during and after the procedure. Following the lifestyle elements of the Healthy Heart Plan will help you stay in shape in the event of surgery.

- -

➜ **Additional resources:**

Mayo Clinic
www.mayoclinic.com

American Heart Association
www.heart.org

National Heart, Lung, and Blood Institute
www.nhlbi.nih.gov

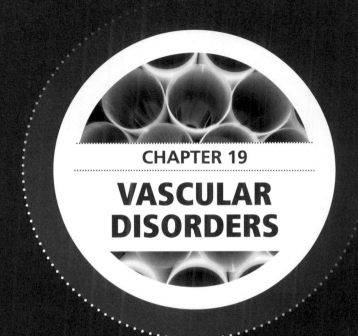

CHAPTER 19

VASCULAR DISORDERS

Your heart isn't the only part of your body where atherosclerosis, high blood pressure and high cholesterol can take a toll. If you have blocked or narrowed arteries in your heart, you have an increased risk of vascular disease. The opposite also is true: If you have vascular disease, you have an increased risk of heart disease.

Narrowed arteries in your heart can lead to chest pain and progress to a heart attack, and the effects elsewhere in your body can be just as detrimental. Narrowed arteries to your limbs, brain, kidneys or lungs can become serious health problems. Fortunately, taking simple steps — even walking just a few minutes several times a day — can have a big effect on your vascular health. Find out how tailoring the Healthy Heart Plan to vascular disease can work for you.

" I notice that when I walk, I'm much more comfortable. My blood pressure goes down. And I discovered that if I don't walk, I don't feel as good. I get cramps in my legs."

JoAn

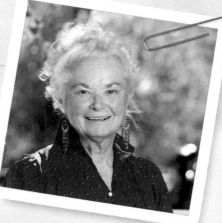

Diagnosis: Peripheral artery disease

Event: Normally, a little leg pain wouldn't keep JoAn from hitting the dance floor — she went out polka or swing dancing two or three times a week. One night, however, her leg hurt so much that she went to the hospital, concerned she might have a blood clot. Years earlier, she'd developed a clot after surgery. Testing ruled out a clot, but an ache in her right leg continued to bother her for weeks. Finally, during a physical exam, JoAn's doctor felt her feet and observed, "One foot is colder than the other. I think it's an artery problem." JoAn was diagnosed with peripheral artery disease and referred to a vascular surgeon. Instead of surgery, he suggested that she begin a walking program of at least 30 minutes a day.

Outcome: JoAn says the walking has made a big difference. She bought a treadmill to use during the winter — and, at age 84, she's still dancing. She met her new husband, Eddie, at a dance, and is busier than ever. "I work harder as a farm wife than I did running two inns," says JoAn, who used to manage two bed-and-breakfast inns. "I'm anxious to live a long time now that I just got married."

High blood pressure (hypertension)

As you've already learned in Chapter 14, your blood pressure measures how much pressure your blood exerts on your blood vessel walls as it circulates through your body. High blood pressure can be dangerous to any blood vessel in your body.

If the pressure increases on a blood vessel wall, the risk of injury to that vessel increases. Your blood vessels can bulge and weaken. The pressure can increase to the point your blood vessels can tear or rupture, a condition called dissection.

Your kidneys play a pivotal role in the way your body controls your blood pressure. If the arteries to your kidneys narrow, it can cause high blood pressure to develop or worsen. The good news is that treatment to open the arteries to your kidneys, such as using a balloon and stent to hold the vessel open, can improve your blood pressure control and reduce your need for medications.

Another blood vessel where high pressure can be particularly dangerous is in the arteries of your lungs (pulmonary arteries). Pulmonary hypertension begins when tiny arteries in your lungs, called pulmonary arteries, become narrowed or destroyed. This makes it harder for blood to flow through your lungs, which raises pressure within the arteries in your lungs. As the pressure builds, your heart's lower right chamber (right ventricle) must work harder to pump blood through your lungs, eventually causing your heart muscle to weaken.

Diseases of the aorta

The aorta is a large blood vessel that transports blood from your heart to the rest of your body. If your aorta becomes diseased, you can develop a bulging weakened spot on the aorta called an aneurysm.

An aneurysm is a weak spot in the vascular wall that forms a balloon-like bulge that may grow larger over time and potentially rupture. Internal bleeding from the rupture is potentially life-threatening.

Aneurysms can develop anywhere along the aorta, but most commonly occur in the lower part of the aorta in your abdomen (abdominal aortic aneurysm). When they occur in the upper part of the aorta, they're called thoracic aortic aneurysms.

Aortic aneurysms often don't have any signs or symptoms. Although doctors aren't often sure of the exact cause of an aortic aneurysm, causes can include damage to the aorta from tobacco use, high blood pressure, an infection or inflammation in the aortic wall, an inherited condition, or an injury to the chest.

Who needs to be screened for aortic aneurysm?

Because aortic aneurysms don't often show signs or symptoms, they can be tricky to diagnose. Rather, researchers have determined it's best to screen at-risk populations. Abdominal aortic aneurysm screening is recommended for:

✔ Anyone age 60 or older who has risk factors for developing an aneurysm, such as smoking or a family history of aortic aneurysm

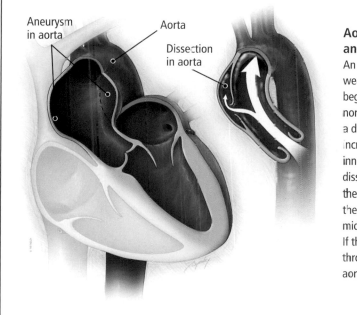

Aneurysm in aorta

Aorta

Dissection in aorta

Aortic aneurysm and dissection

An aortic aneurysm occurs when a weak spot in the wall of your aorta begins to bulge. (The outline of a normal aorta is shown at left with a dashed line.) Having an aneurysm increases the risk of a tear in the inner lining of the aorta, called aortic dissection. Blood surges through the tear into the middle layer of the aorta, causing the inner and middle layers to separate (dissect). If the blood-filled channel ruptures through the outside aortic wall, aortic dissection is usually fatal.

- ✓ Men ages 65 to 75 who have ever smoked cigarettes
- ✓ Men age 60 and older with a family history of abdominal aortic aneurysm

Screening for abdominal aortic aneurysm is usually performed by an ultrasound of your abdomen.

Screening for thoracic aortic aneurysm is recommended for people who have a family history of the condition, or have a connective tissue disease, such as Marfan syndrome. Screening tests may include a chest X-ray, echocardiogram, CT scan or magnetic resonance angiography (MRA). These tests are described in Chapter 21: Common diagnostic tests.

Your doctor can help you determine how frequently you may need screening exams for aortic aneurysm. You may need regular ultrasound exams if you have a family history of aortic aneurysm.

Complications of aortic aneurysm

+ **Aortic dissection or rupture.** An aneurysm can become large enough to tear the wall of your aorta (dissection) or rupture. An aortic dissection or rupture is a medical emergency.

Marfan syndrome and aortic disease

If you've been diagnosed with Marfan syndrome, a genetic condition that affects your body's connective tissue, you should be especially concerned about the health of your aorta. People who have Marfan syndrome are more likely to develop an aortic aneurysm or dissection. Be sure to talk to your doctor about regular echocardiograms and other screening tests to make sure your aorta hasn't developed any weaknesses or bulging spots.

If you have sudden, extreme pain in your chest or abdomen, pain that radiates to your back or legs, weakness or fainting, seek emergency medical care immediately.

+ **Blood clots.** Small blood clots can develop in the area of an abdominal aortic aneurysm. If a blood clot breaks loose from the inside wall of an aneurysm and blocks a blood vessel in your body, it can cause pain or block the blood flow to the legs, toes, kidneys or abdominal organs.

Peripheral artery disease

If atherosclerosis develops in another blood vessel, such as the arteries in your legs or arms, it can limit the amount of oxygenated blood that reaches those parts of your body. This condition is known as peripheral artery disease (PAD). The condition can cause leg pain severe enough to discourage you from being active, or if left untreated, cause circulation problems that may make it difficult for wounds to heal.

Symptoms of PAD

- ✔ Painful cramping in your hip, thigh or calf muscles after activity, such as walking or climbing stairs
- ✔ Leg numbness or weakness
- ✔ Coldness in a lower leg or foot, especially when compared with the other leg
- ✔ Sores on your toes, feet or legs that won't heal
- ✔ Hair loss or slower hair growth on your feet and legs

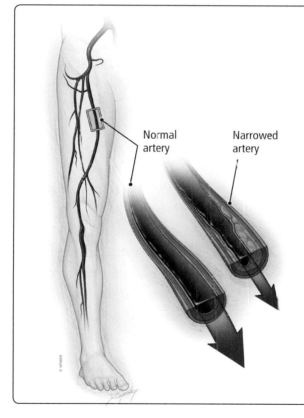

Normal artery

Narrowed artery

Development of peripheral artery disease

In normal circulation (the artery shown at left), blood easily travels through arteries down your legs to supply your tissues with oxygen and other nutrients, and returns to your heart and lungs upward through your veins (see Chapter 13). In peripheral artery disease, atherosclerosis narrows the blood vessels in your legs (the artery shown at right), making it harder for adequate blood supply to reach the tissues in your legs. This can lead to pain while exercising or at rest. Worse, a lack of adequate blood flow can mean wounds on your legs and feet can't heal as quickly as they would with normal circulation. Wounds can become infected and, if left untreated, lead to gangrene that can require amputation.

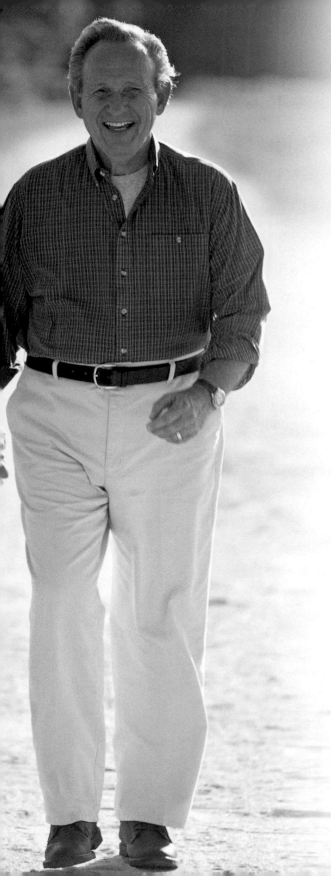

- ✔ Slower growth of your toenails
- ✔ Shiny skin on your legs
- ✔ No pulse or a weak pulse in your legs or feet
- ✔ A change in the color of your legs

If PAD goes untreated, the pain in your affected limb will worsen as the blood flow becomes more limited. Eventually, your limb may receive so little oxygenated blood that you develop a condition called critical limb ischemia (CLI). This condition begins as open sores that don't heal, an injury, or an infection of your feet or legs. CLI occurs when such injuries or infections progress and can cause tissue death (gangrene). Gangrene sometimes requires amputation of the affected arm or leg.

Who should be screened for peripheral artery disease?

Screening for PAD in certain high-risk groups, even without symptoms, is recommended by some organizations, including the American Heart Association and the American College of Cardiology. Your doctor may recommend PAD screening tests even if you don't have symptoms if you are:

- ✔ Older than age 50 and have a history of diabetes or smoking

- Older than age 65 and your doctor feels that finding PAD would change your treatment

The test to diagnose PAD is called an ankle-brachial index. This is a non-invasive test that measures your blood pressure at your ankle using a special blood pressure cuff and a Doppler ultrasound device to monitor the blood flow through the blood vessels in your ankle. The blood pressure measurements are compared with the blood pressure at your arm.

Be cautious of routine screenings promoted by for-profit clinics. Screening for PAD should be done as part of an evaluation with your doctor.

Walking for PAD

Given it might be painful for you to walk if you have PAD, you may find it surprising that walking is one of the best lifestyle changes you can make to improve your condition. The key is to start out slowly and gradually increase your distance and speed.

Talk to your doctor about starting at an appropriate pace and time limit for your condition. You may only be able

Specialist focus:

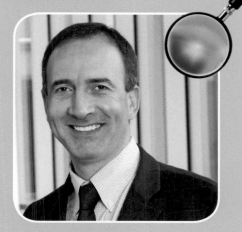

Issam D. Moussa, M.D., is an expert in cardiac and vascular disease at Mayo Clinic.

Many people think that leg pain or an inability to walk is a result of old age or arthritis. But it could well be because of plaques in the arteries in the legs. If you have leg pain … have it checked.

to walk slowly for a few minutes at first. Don't be discouraged — stick with the program. It may take up to two to six months for you to notice improvement in your condition. Make sure you wear footwear that's supportive and

Vascular health and sex

Following the Healthy Heart Plan can have greater benefits than a reduced risk of heart disease. For men, atherosclerosis and high blood pressure can also affect blood vessels in the penis, causing erectile dysfunction (ED). Because the arteries to the penis are narrower than those near your heart, ED may show up three to five years before life-threatening problems, such as heart attack and stroke.

ED is a common condition — it affects about 1 out of 5 men. Although there are medications to treat ED, following a heart-healthy lifestyle may reduce the need for those medications, or may help those medications work better. If you're already taking ED medications and they become less effective, "that should be a sign that ... you need to take care of your lifestyle," says Stephen L. Kopecky, M.D., a cardiologist at Mayo Clinic. "Men don't sit around worrying about heart disease, but they do worry about not being able to have sex," he says.

In addition to diet, exercise and good quality sleep, statins can be particularly effective in improving vascular health for men who have ED. The earlier you start the Healthy Heart Plan, the more your risk of developing heart disease decreases. For partners of men who have ED, the condition can present an opportunity to talk about taking steps to prevent heart disease and improve ED symptoms.

Less is known about cardiovascular disease and women's sexual health. High blood pressure can reduce blood flow to the vagina, leading to a decrease in sexual desire, vaginal dryness or difficulty achieving orgasm. Talk to your doctor if you're having these troubles.

appropriate for walking. Go as far as you can, rest, and then walk some more. You may find that four to six short walks a day might be your best option. Eventually, you'll be able to walk longer at one time. If the circulation in your legs is poor, check your feet after each walk for any sores, cuts or blisters. Wear shoes that fit comfortably without any pressure points.

Keep a log of how far you walked and how long it took you. Make a note of any pains you felt and how intense the pain was on a scale of 1 to 10.

Don't forget about the arteries to your head and neck

Just as arteries in your heart and limbs can be affected by atherosclerosis, so can the arteries in your neck (carotid and vertebral arteries). This can limit blood flow to your brain, a condition called cerebrovascular disease.

Cerebrovascular disease can cause a stroke, or a transient ischemic attack (TIA), a condition that's similar to a stroke but without permanent damage to your brain.

Similar treatments for coronary artery disease can be helpful for cerebrovascular disease. Your doctor may prescribe many of the same medications to control your condition. Just as stents and surgery are used for coronary artery disease, doctors may recommend similar procedures to help blood flow up to your brain. As with any type of atherosclerosis, living a heart-healthy lifestyle also reduces your risk of a stroke.

What are the symptoms of a stroke?

If you're having a stroke, you may not realize it. To a bystander, someone having a stroke may just look unaware or confused. People who are having a stroke have the best chance if someone around them recognizes the symptoms and acts quickly to call for emergency help.

The symptoms of stroke are distinct because they happen quickly:

+ Sudden numbness or weakness of the face, arm or leg (especially on one side of the body)

+ Sudden confusion, trouble speaking or understanding speech

+ Sudden trouble seeing in one or both eyes

+ Sudden trouble walking, dizziness, loss of balance or coordination

+ Sudden severe headache with no known cause

Call for emergency medical assistance if you or someone else has these symptoms.

Adapting the Healthy Heart Plan to vascular disease

1 **Quit tobacco use and avoid secondhand smoke.** Although quitting tobacco use and avoiding secondhand smoke are important for anyone, they are especially important for people who have PAD or an aortic aneurysm. Tobacco use and second-hand smoke damage the walls of your arteries, making the aorta more vulnerable to weakening and ruptur-ing. This damage can also make it more likely that plaques will form in the smaller vessels of your legs and arms, worsening PAD.

2 **Find out if you have exercise or weightlifting restrictions.** While exercise is helpful in keeping your blood vessels healthy, you may need to follow some exercise restrictions if you have an aneurysm that requires more than medical monitoring. If you have an aortic aneurysm, your doctor may recommend you not play any competi-tive sports or lift heavy weights (no more than 50 pounds).

3 **Modify your walking program.** The aches and pains that come with PAD may discourage you from exercising, but with your doctor's OK, keep at it. Walking is one of the best exercise options for people with PAD because it helps blood flow through the vessels in your legs. Your doctor may recommend breaking up your daily activity into shorter walking sessions of about 10 minutes to minimize your discomfort.

4 **Reach for a low LDL cholesterol target.** Although the target LDL goal for many people with PAD is less than 100 milligrams per deciliter, or mg/dL, your doctor may discuss reaching an even lower goal if you have PAD. If you have diabetes, high blood pressure, high cholesterol, or you smoke, your doctor may recommend a goal of 70 mg/dL.

5 **Know your family history.** Aortic aneurysms often run in families. You should find out if your parents or siblings have ever had an aortic aneurysm, aortic dissection, a bicuspid aortic valve or inherited conditions such as Marfan syndrome. Similarly, if you're diagnosed with an aortic aneurysm, talk to your family members about getting screened for the condition. PAD can run in families as well. When you're being screened for heart disease, try to remember if any of your family members had peripheral artery disease in addition to other heart conditions.

6 **Protect your feet if you have peripheral artery disease.** Because peripheral artery disease can limit blood flow through your legs and feet, it may take wounds longer to heal, leaving you prone to infections. Try to avoid injuries to your feet by wearing shoes that fit well and cover your entire foot. Avoid situations where your foot might get injured.

7 **Keep up with follow-up appointments.** If your doctor recommends medical monitoring for an aortic aneurysm, be sure to make it to every appointment for checkups. Medical monitoring is not the same as doing nothing — your doctor will need to make sure your aneurysm isn't growing. If your aneurysm is growing, the sooner your doctor finds out, the quicker he or she can act to repair the damaged portion of your aorta and reduce your risk of rupture, dissection or death.

- -

➜ **Additional resources:**

Mayo Clinic
www.mayoclinic.com

Pulmonary hypertension association
www.phassociation.org

National Marfan Foundation
www.marfan.org

National Heart, Lung, and Blood Institute
www.nhlbi.nih.gov

CHAPTER 20

CONGENITAL HEART DISEASE

Receiving a diagnosis of congenital heart disease, either as a child or as an adult, can feel devastating. You may be fearful about a reduction in your quality of life, or about the medical care you may need for the rest of your life. Fortunately, medical advances have made it so diagnosis of a congenital heart disease doesn't need to be cause for panic.

Congenital heart disease occurs when you have problems in your heart that are present at birth. The defect may be diagnosed while you are still in the womb, shortly after birth, during childhood, or sometimes not even until adulthood. Some forms of congenital heart disease are obvious and easily diagnosed, but others may go undetected for many years until signs and symptoms develop.

> " It's scary to think about what could have happened. I know I'm lucky to be alive. "

David

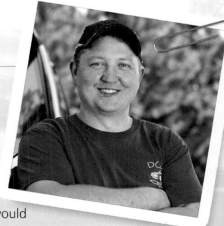

Diagnosis: Coarctation of the aorta, bicuspid aortic valve, aortic aneurysm

Event: Born with a heart defect called coarctation of the aorta (a narrowing of part of the aorta) and an abnormal heart valve, David had surgery at age three and a half. His mom, Ruth, recalls, "When David was little, he kept telling me, 'Mommy, my legs hurt.' He would also get chest pain and pound on his chest." After the surgery, David recovered quickly. His legs stopped hurting, he grew 3½ inches in one year, and his weight rebounded from the low of eight pounds he had reached.

After graduating from high school, however, David no longer received regular medical care. At age 29, he agreed to participate in a research study. Routine tests showed that part of his aorta was massively enlarged to more than twice the normal size — the aorta could burst (rupture) at any time. Furthermore, his aortic valve was leaking severely. Although David felt fine and had no symptoms, he needed urgent open heart surgery to prevent a fatal rupture.

Outcome: David had surgery to replace his enlarged aorta and the leaky valve. Now, he's back to working as a mechanic. He makes sure that he keeps up with regular follow-up visits and had his son checked for heart problems. He enjoys fishing with his son and working on his truck. "I'm just a regular guy."

Many heart defects that are diagnosed in adulthood need only medical monitoring or medications to keep the condition well managed. If you need surgery or other procedures to manage a heart defect, your doctor can help you decide what course of treatment may be the best option for you.

Causes and misconceptions

No one's sure what causes congenital heart disease, but the defect develops in the womb while your heart is still forming. Some heart defects have a genetic connection, while others might be caused by medications taken during pregnancy. Smoking, alcohol use or use of illegal drugs during pregnancy also may play a role.

Common types of congenital heart disease include holes in the walls of the heart chambers (septal defects), narrowing of the heart's main artery (coarctation of aorta), malformations of the heart that cause oxygen-poor blood to flow out to the body (cyanotic heart disease, such as tetralogy of Fallot — a combination of four heart defects) and a problem with the placement of the heart's arteries (transposition of great arteries).

It's possible that a heart defect you were born with does not cause signs or symptoms until you're an adult. Some defects are so mild that they're difficult to detect. But the defects that never caused problems before may start to do so now as you age.

A common misconception about congenital heart disease is that once the defect has been treated, it's repaired for life. But some adults may find that the problems arise later in life, even after childhood treatment. This is because heart defects are seldom cured — they are often repaired, so heart function is improved, but your heart is often not completely normal.

There are many reasons why signs and symptoms from heart defects can re-emerge in adults. In some cases, the treatment you received in childhood may have been successful initially, but the problem worsens later in life. It's also possible that a defect in your heart, which wasn't serious enough to repair when you were a child, has worsened and now requires treatment.

Complications of childhood surgeries to repair congenital heart defects can

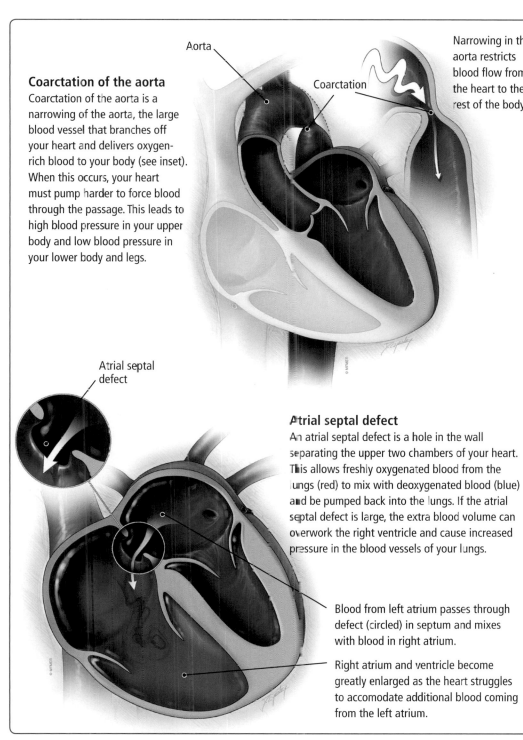

Coarctation of the aorta

Coarctation of the aorta is a narrowing of the aorta, the large blood vessel that branches off your heart and delivers oxygen-rich blood to your body (see inset). When this occurs, your heart must pump harder to force blood through the passage. This leads to high blood pressure in your upper body and low blood pressure in your lower body and legs.

Aorta

Coarctation

Narrowing in the aorta restricts blood flow from the heart to the rest of the body.

Atrial septal defect

Atrial septal defect

An atrial septal defect is a hole in the wall separating the upper two chambers of your heart. This allows freshly oxygenated blood from the lungs (red) to mix with deoxygenated blood (blue) and be pumped back into the lungs. If the atrial septal defect is large, the extra blood volume can overwork the right ventricle and cause increased pressure in the blood vessels of your lungs.

Blood from left atrium passes through defect (circled) in septum and mixes with blood in right atrium.

Right atrium and ventricle become greatly enlarged as the heart struggles to accomodate additional blood coming from the left atrium.

occur later in life. Many treatments may leave scar tissue behind in your heart muscle that increases the chance of an abnormal heart rhythm (arrhythmia) or a problem with blood flow through your heart.

Because these complications can arise at any time, it's important to schedule regular appointments with a doctor who has expertise in treating congenital heart disease.

Symptoms

Although congenital heart disease is often diagnosed early in an individual's life, the signs and symptoms may not show up until much later. And the symptoms may recur years after a defect is treated. Typical symptoms of congenital heart disease that you may experience as an adult include:

- Abnormal heart rhythms (arrhythmias)
- A bluish tint to the skin (cyanosis)
- Shortness of breath
- Tiring quickly upon exertion
- Dizziness or fainting
- Swelling of body tissue or organs (edema)

Complications

+ **Abnormal heart rhythms (arrhythmias)**. Heart rhythm problems are common in people with congenital heart disease as they age. The heart defect may interfere with normal electrical impulses, or previous corrective surgery has left scar tissue. In some people, the arrhythmias can become severe, causing shortness of breath, fainting or cardiac arrest.

+ **Heart infections (endocarditis).** Your heart's chambers and valves are lined by a thin membrane called the endocardium. Endocarditis is an infection of this inner lining. Some defects interrupt the smooth flow of blood in your heart, making it easier for bacteria to collect in the lining. Left untreated, endocarditis can damage your heart valves, trigger a stroke, or lead to death.

+ **Stroke.** Some congenital heart defects increase your risk of stroke due to an abnormal connection in the heart allowing a blood clot from a vein to travel to your brain. Certain heart arrhythmias also can increase your chance of blood clot formation leading to a stroke.

- **Heart failure.** Heart failure means your heart can't pump enough blood to meet your body's needs. Some types of congenital heart disease can lead to heart failure.

- **Pulmonary hypertension.** This type of high blood pressure affects only the arteries in your lungs. Congenital heart disease may cause more blood to flow to the lungs, gradually increasing pressure. If not caught early, permanent damage to the lungs can occur.

- **Heart valve problems.** In some types of congenital heart disease, the heart valves are abnormal. An abnormal valve may not open properly or leak.

Diagnosis and treatment

If you were diagnosed with a heart defect as a child, make sure your doctor knows about your medical history. You will likely need periodic checks of your heart's function and structure to make sure it's healthy and to prevent complications. Talk to your doctor about how often you'll need follow-up appointments. Monitoring your

Specialist focus:

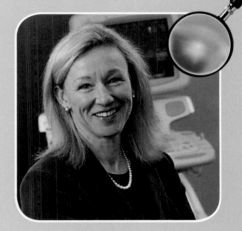

Heidi M. Connolly, M.D., is an expert in congenital heart disease at Mayo Clinic.

If you have congenital heart disease, you should know what condition you have, what procedures you may have had, and what medications you take. You should ideally carry a document that outlines this, as well as contact information for quick access to medical records.

You should have regular follow-ups with a congenital cardiologist, and consult with the cardiologist before having a major procedure, operation or pregnancy.

heart disease is not the same as doing nothing — you'll need regular evaluations to keep track of your condition in case you'll require medications or surgery.

Medications can make sure your condition doesn't get worse, or help prevent other heart conditions such as coronary artery disease. You may need medications to lower blood pressure or cholesterol, to control your heart's rhythm, or to treat heart failure.

If your heart defect is severe, you may need surgery, both as a child and an adult, to repair the defect. In rare cases, you may need a heart transplant if the defect can't be repaired surgically or if heart function deteriorates.

Adapting the Healthy Heart Plan to congenital heart disease

1 **Know your medical history.** If you have congenital heart disease, it's imperative that you tell your doctor about previous and current treatments, including medications and surgeries. Your doctor will want to know how you responded to medications you've taken

in the past. Your previous surgeries may give clues as to how the structure of your heart has changed and what problems could develop in the future.

Because some heart defects can be hereditary, it's important to know the medical history of your parents, siblings and children. Ask your doctor if family members should also be screened for heart defects.

2 **Understand exercise limitations, if you have any.** If you have congenital heart disease, it's important that you talk to your doctor before starting an exercise program. Your heart defect may restrict the type of activities you can do, but you will likely be able to be physically active. Depending on your condition, your doctor may recommend that you avoid competitive sports, weightlifting or vigorous aerobic exercise.

3 **Ask your doctor about preventive antibiotics.** Most heart defects, especially those that affect your heart's valves, carry a risk of infection. For many years, doctors recommended taking antibiotics before certain medical and dental procedures for almost all people who had congenital heart disease. This has changed, however. Many people who have a heart defect no longer need preventive antibiotics. Ask your doctor if you'll need to take antibiotics before having medical or dental procedures.

4 **Have a plan for emergency medical care.** Should you have a medical emergency, it's important for emergency personnel to know you have congenital heart disease and what medications you may take or surgeries you had. Consider wearing a medical identification bracelet or carrying a card in your wallet that details your heart condition and treatments. Make sure your cardiologist is alerted to changes in your condition.

5 **Understand the importance of sleep disorders.** As with any heart condition, the signs and symptoms of your heart defect can worsen if you have a sleep disorder, such as sleep apnea. Sleep disorders can be particularly dangerous with congenital heart disease. That's because it can cause low oxygen levels, high blood pressure and heart rhythm problems that may worsen your heart function or cause sudden death.

6 **Talk to your doctor about family planning.** Most women who have congenital heart disease can have a successful pregnancy with proper care. If you have a congenital defect, it's important to have a medical exam from a doctor who has expertise in congenital heart disease before becoming pregnant. Ask if there are special risks to you or your baby, such as the risk of the baby inheriting your heart defect. Find out if you can continue your medications during pregnancy.

If you plan to use birth control (contraceptives), talk to your doctor first. Some contraceptives containing estrogen may not be appropriate for women who have increased risk of blood clots.

- -

➜ Additional resources:

Mayo Clinic
www.mayoclinic.com

Adult Congenital Heart Association
www.achaheart.org

National Heart, Lung, and Blood, Institute
www.nhlbi.nih.gov

PART 4

SUPPORT
YOUR PLAN

You learned the basics of the Mayo Clinic Healthy Heart Plan earlier in the book. This section provides you with additional support, if you need it. Remember that 80 percent of heart disease is preventable, and making healthy changes in your life is easier and more enjoyable than you may think.

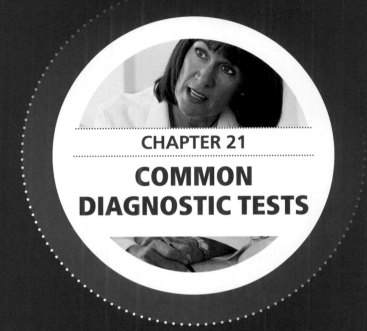

CHAPTER 21

COMMON DIAGNOSTIC TESTS

Maybe you suspect something is wrong — say you find yourself winded after a single flight of stairs or you have occasional chest pains — and you've scheduled a medical appointment to have it checked out. Or perhaps you're simply wondering what kinds of tests will be used for your heart during a routine physical exam. It's both helpful and reassuring to know what to expect when your doctor checks your heart health.

The tests your doctor may use to assess your heart health will depend on your age and risk factors for heart disease, and whether you have any signs or symptoms of heart disease. Your doctor will likely perform a physical exam and ask about your personal and family medical history before doing any testing.

Here are the tests typically used to study heart health and function.

Blood tests

The makeup of your blood can offer clues about your heart health. This typically requires a small amount of your blood to be drawn and tested for substances that may indicate you are at increased risk of heart disease.

Before you have any blood tests, be sure to ask your doctor if you'll need to make any special preparations. You may need to fast overnight or temporarily stop taking some medications.

As you've read in previous chapters, the cholesterol and triglyceride levels in your blood provide key information about heart health. Too much

low-density lipoprotein (LDL) cholesterol or too little high-density lipoprotein (HDL) cholesterol puts you at greater risk of atherosclerosis — the accumulation of fatty deposits in your blood vessels. A high level of triglycerides may contribute to atherosclerosis and can also be a sign of poorly managed diabetes.

A fasting plasma glucose test measures your blood sugar levels and can help your doctor determine if you have diabetes or are at risk of developing the condition. Having diabetes increases your risk of heart disease.

Blood tests can also check your level of the thyroid hormone. High levels of this hormone can increase your risk of cardiovascular disease. Elevated levels of certain proteins, such as troponin and creatine kinase-MB, that are released from injured or dying heart muscle tissues also may be signs of muscle damage resulting from a heart attack.

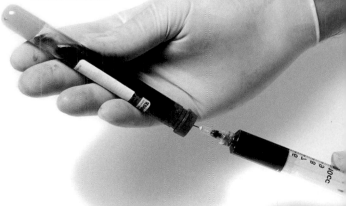

Other blood tests that may be used for diagnosis, treatment and management of heart disease include:

+ **C-reactive protein (CRP).** The presence of this protein in your blood can indicate inflammation, a key part of developing atherosclerosis. Measuring CRP alone won't reveal your risk of heart disease, but factoring in these test results with other blood test results helps create an overall picture of your heart health.

+ **Fibrinogen.** This is a protein that helps blood clot. Having too much fibrinogen in your blood may mean atherosclerosis. It may also worsen existing injury to your artery walls.

+ **Homocysteine.** Your body uses this substance to make protein and to build and maintain tissue. But too much homocysteine may increase your risk of stroke, heart disease and peripheral artery disease.

+ **Lipoprotein (a).** This type of LDL cholesterol is determined by your genes and isn't generally affected by your lifestyle. Your doctor might

order this test if you already have atherosclerosis or heart disease but appear to have normal cholesterol levels, or if you have a strong family history of heart disease.

+ **Natriuretic peptides.** These proteins are helpful in diagnosing heart failure, but must be considered along with your signs and symptoms and results of other tests.

Electrocardiogram

For an electrocardiogram (ECG), a technician places electrodes on your arms, legs and chest to record the electrical impulses that make your heart beat.

An ECG can help your doctor detect irregularities in your heart's rhythm and structure. You may have an ECG while you're at rest or while you're exercising (stress electrocardiogram).

The few minutes that a standard ECG is recording may not capture heartbeat irregularity that comes and goes. In this case, your doctor may recommend a Holter monitor, a portable device that you wear to record a continuous ECG, usually for 24 to 72 hours.

For sporadic rhythm problems, you can wear a portable ECG device called an event recorder for several weeks or longer. You attach it to your body and activate it only when you experience symptoms. This lets your doctor track your heart rhythm at the time of your symptoms, to help make a diagnosis.

Stress tests

A stress test helps measure how well your heart muscle is functioning and whether it's receiving enough blood.

The test results may help your doctor evaluate symptoms such as chest pain or shortness of breath that develop when you're physically active.

If you've had a heart attack, your doctor may order a stress test to check the damage to your heart and determine if you need additional treatment.

Stress tests are sometimes recommended before you begin a program of vigorous exercise, particularly if you have cardiovascular risk factors.

Electrocardiogram
An electrocardiogram monitors your heart rhythm for problems. Electrodes are taped to your chest to record your heart's electrical signals, which cause your heart to beat. The signals are shown as waves on an attached computer monitor or printer.

Exercise stress test

A technician places electrodes on your chest, similar to a standard ECG, and wraps a blood pressure cuff on your arm. You then walk on a treadmill while an ECG records how your heart rate responds to an increasing workload. As the speed and grade of the treadmill is gradually increased and the workout becomes more demanding, your heart rate increases.

The health care professional overseeing the test will be monitoring factors such as heart rate and blood pressure. For people who can't walk on a treadmill, other forms of exercise, such as pedaling a stationary bicycle or doing arm exercises, are sometimes used.

Exercise stress tests are often combined with imaging tests that produce pictures of the heart muscle to determine if it's getting enough blood.

Nonexercise stress test

A nonexercise (pharmacological) stress test is used for individuals who can't

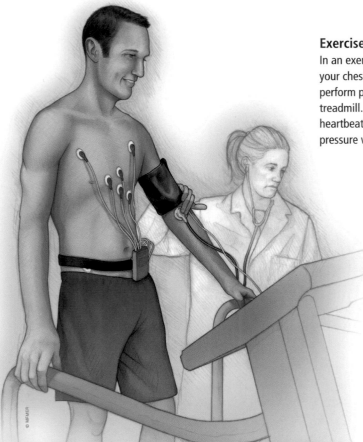

Exercise stress test

In an exercise stress test, electrodes are taped to your chest to detect your heart's rhythm as you perform physical activity, such as walking on a treadmill. A nurse or technician will watch your heartbeat on a monitor and check your blood pressure while you exercise.

exercise due to conditions such as arthritis. Your doctor may also order this test if you have heart rhythm problems, which could make the results of an exercise stress test inconclusive.

For the test, a medication is injected into your bloodstream that stresses your heart, mimicking the effects of exercise. The effects of the medication are observed with imaging tests.

If either test indicates that your heart was unaffected by stress, it's likely that your heart will function properly when you exercise. If the test reveals problems, the results can help in setting up exercise limits and developing a specialized fitness program. If the ECG from the test shows abnormal patterns, your doctor may order additional tests or prescribe medications to improve blood flow to your heart.

Imaging tests

Actual images of the heart may be necessary that allow doctors to see tissue damage or structural abnormalities of certain conditions. Some techniques can also reveal areas of the heart that may not be functioning properly.

Chest X-ray

An X-ray machine produces a small burst of radiation that passes through your body and forms a clear image on photographic film or a digital recording plate that's been positioned on the other side. A chest X-ray generates a picture of your heart, lungs and large blood vessels. It can reveal if your heart is enlarged — a sign of some forms of heart disease. The X-ray can also reveal fluid buildup in or around your lungs, a sign of heart failure.

Echocardiogram

An echocardiogram uses ultrasound technology to generate detailed images of your heart's structure and function. A device called a transducer, which is gently pressed against your skin, transmits sound waves and collects the echoes reflected off tissues and fluids in your body. A computer uses information from the transducer to create moving images on a video monitor.

This commonly used test allows your doctor to see how well your heart is beating and pumping blood. It can also be used to identify abnormalities in the heart muscle and valves, and determine if your heart has been damaged by a heart attack. An echocardiogram

© MFMER

A warning on walk-in heart scans

Some walk-in clinics may advertise quick heart scans that look for calcium buildup in your arteries, which may show you're at risk of having a heart attack. However, these scans are not recommended for most people without consultation from their doctors. Be cautious.

can also check the pumping function of your heart (ejection fraction) and fluid build-up around the heart. For more on the ejection fraction, see page 142.

If more detailed views of your heart are necessary, your doctor may recommend a transesophageal ultrasound. For this exam, your throat is numbed and you swallow a long, flexible tube containing a tiny transducer. The transducer is guided down your throat and, when in position close to the heart, transmits images.

Echocardiogram

An echocardiogram generates images to check how your heart's chambers and valves are pumping blood through your heart. A technician lightly presses a transducer against your chest to produce the images using ultrasound technology. Electrodes taped to your chest check your heart rhythm. An echocardiogram can help your doctor diagnose heart conditions and identify abnormalities or damage in the heart muscle or valves.

Cardiac catheterization

Cardiac catheterization (coronary angiogram) begins with a short tube (sheath) inserted into a vein or artery in your leg or arm. A hollow, flexible and longer tube (guide catheter) is then inserted into the sheath. Aided by X-ray images on a monitor, your doctor threads the guide catheter through the artery until it reaches your heart.

With the catheter in place, your doctor can measure pressures in your heart chambers, and inject dye into the heart. The dye sharpens what can be seen on an X-ray, which helps your doctor to better see the blood flowing through your heart, blood vessels and valves to check for abnormalities.

If necessary, your doctor can perform procedures such as angioplasty and stent placement during your coronary angiogram. Doctors can sometimes use the procedure to repair or replace damaged heart valves, eliminating the need for open heart surgery.

Cardiac computerized tomography

Cardiac computerized tomography (CT) scans can show the size and function of your heart muscle and check for certain valve problems. For the test, you lie on a table inside a doughnut-shaped machine. An X-ray tube inside the machine rotates around your body and collects images of your heart and chest.

A cardiac CT scan may be used to measure the amount of calcium in the walls of your coronary arteries, which supply your heart with blood. The calcium may indicate that you have coronary artery disease, the leading cause of heart attacks.

The procedure is also often used to check for blood clots in your heart and lungs or a tear in your aorta (dissection). Because these conditions are life-threatening, the procedure is commonly used in the emergency department of hospitals to evaluate people with chest pain.

Cardiac magnetic resonance imaging

For cardiac magnetic resonance imaging (MRI), you lie on a table inside a long tube-like machine that produces a magnetic field. The magnetic field aligns atomic particles in some of your cells. When radio waves are broadcast toward these particles, they produce signals that vary according to the type of tissue they are.

Cardiac MRI images of your heart are created from these signals, which your doctor will use to help determine the cause of a heart condition. These scans are helpful in diagnosing unexplained heart failure, checking for inflammation of the heart (myocarditis) and monitoring congenital heart disease.

Taking your blood pressure

A blood pressure test measures the pressure in your arteries as your heart pumps. You might have a blood pressure test as a part of a routine doctor visit or as screening for high blood pressure (hypertension). Many people, such as those with high blood pressure, do their own blood pressure tests at home so that they can better track their health.

In the doctor's office

During a routine doctor visit, your blood pressure may be measured by a nurse or technician either manually or with the help of a digital machine.

The test is performed best while you're seated in a chair in the examining room. Your arm should be supported and resting on a table, at about the level of your heart. Both of your feet should be flat on the floor and your back supported by the chair. During the test, you shouldn't attempt to talk or move your arm.

The nurse or technician will wrap an inflatable cuff around the top part of your arm. The cuff is attached to a digital display, a dial or a device that looks similar to a thermometer.

The cuff is gently inflated to momentarily stop blood flow through the artery in your arm, then quickly deflated to reopen blood flow.

During this process, the digital machine automatically reads your pulse to figure out your blood pressure. If done manually, the nurse or technician reads your pulse with the help of a stethoscope. See Chapter 7 for information on blood pressure target numbers.

Your doctor will likely require two to three blood pressure readings each at two or more separate visits before diagnosing you with high blood pressure. This is because blood pressure normally varies throughout the day and from day to day. By taking multiple readings over a span of time, your doctor will know that your blood pressure stays consistently high.

If you have high blood pressure, your doctor may recommend routine tests, such as a urine test (urinalysis), blood tests and an electrocardiogram (ECG). Your doctor may also recommend additional tests, such as a cholesterol test, to check for more signs of heart disease.

At home

If you have high blood pressure, it may be necessary to monitor your blood pressure at home. The record of home test results that you compile often is a vital asset to treating your condition.

An automatic blood pressure monitor is often used for home monitoring. Find a comfortable place to sit with good back support at a table or desk. When you're ready to take your blood pressure, sit quietly for three to five minutes beforehand. Position yourself in the same way that you sit for an office visit, with your arm stretched out, palm upward.

Place the cuff on your bare upper arm one inch above the bend of your elbow. Make sure the tubing falls over the front center of your arm so that the sensor is correctly placed. Pull the end of the cuff so that it's evenly tight around your arm. You should place it tight enough so that you can only slip two fingertips under the top edge of the cuff. Make sure your skin doesn't pinch when the cuff inflates.

Wait a moment, then press the button to start. Remain still and quiet as the machine begins measuring.

© MFMER

Taking your blood pressure at home

The American Heart Association and other organizations recommend anyone with high blood pressure to monitor his or her blood pressure at home. Home monitoring can help you keep tabs on your blood pressure in a familiar setting, make certain your medications are working, and alert you and your doctors to potential health complications. You can record your readings in a blood pressure log, whether on paper (see sample below) or electronically, such as in an online personal health record or blood pressure tracker, for example.

Sample blood pressure log

Date	Time	Systolic pressure	Diastolic pressure	Pulse	Medication changes / comments

The cuff will inflate, then slowly deflate while the machine takes your measurement. When the reading is complete, the digital panel displays your blood pressure and pulse. If the monitor doesn't record a reading, reposition the cuff and try again. Rest quietly and wait about one to two minutes before taking another measurement.

Record your numbers, either by writing the information down on paper or by entering it into an electronic record. Some monitors can upload your blood pressure readings directly into a computer or mobile device.

Taking your pulse

When you take your pulse, you feel your heartbeat in one of your arteries. Monitoring your pulse can be helpful, for example, if you want to check your heart rate when you exercise.

To take your own pulse, turn the palm side of your hand up. Put the tips of your index and middle fingers of your opposite hand on your wrist as shown. They should be on the radial artery between your wrist bone and tendon. Apply enough pressure so you can count each beat but don't push too hard. You should feel your pulse. Count the beats for 10 seconds and multiply this number by six. This is your pulse rate.

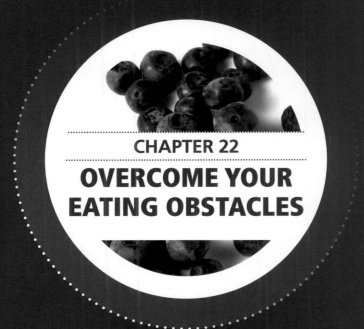

CHAPTER 22

OVERCOME YOUR EATING OBSTACLES

Long-term success with getting healthy sometimes follows a bumpy, uneven path, especially when it comes to adapting to a healthy way of eating. Many obstacles can keep you from reaching your nutritional goals.

Learning to identify potential roadblocks and confront personal temptations is a key part of achieving success. To make it past the rough spots, it's important to have strategies ready to guide your responses as problems arise.

This chapter identifies common nutritional barriers and practical strategies for overcoming them. If you find a strategy that helps you, include it with your overall program.

» Obstacle
I don't have time to make healthy meals.

Having too little time to cook is a common obstacle for many people to eat healthy. Even when meal preparations are rushed, it's possible to find ways to eat healthier. Tasty, nutritious meals don't require a lot of cooking time, but they do require that you plan ahead.

» Strategies
Here are tips to help you eat well on a busy schedule.

+ Plan a week's worth of meals at a time. Make a detailed grocery list to eliminate last-minute trips to the grocery store.

+ Devote time on the weekend to preparing meals for the coming week. Consider making several meals and freezing them in meal-size batches.

+ Remember that healthy meals don't have to be complicated. Serve a fresh salad with fat-free dressing, a whole-grain roll and a piece of fruit.

+ Keep staple ingredients on hand for making basic meals. For example, you can quickly mix together rice, beans and spices for a Tex-Mex casserole.

+ Have family members help in the kitchen. Split up the tasks to save time.

+ On days when you don't have time to make a healthy meal, stop at a deli or grocery store and purchase a healthy sandwich, soup or prepared entree that's low in calories and low in fat.

›› Obstacle
My diet needs a complete overhaul. But I have no idea how to get started.

Even when you know eating certain foods can increase your heart disease risk, it's often tough to change your eating habits. Whether you have years of unhealthy eating under your belt or you simply want to fine-tune your diet, there are eating plans and guidelines that can help you get on track.

The eating plans shown here share things in common. They're based on plant foods that are low in fat and high in fiber, and they're governed by principles of variety, balance and moderation. Certain diets may be designed especially for certain conditions. But any of the following options are considered heart healthy. Your doctor can give you further input on dietary changes that can help you.

›› Strategies
Consider using one of these heart-healthy eating plans as a guideline to get you started.

 ## The Mayo Clinic Diet

Although tailored to help with weight loss, The Mayo Clinic Diet can also be considered a heart-healthy eating approach. With the Mayo Clinic Healthy Weight Pyramid (see page 259) at its core, The Mayo Clinic Diet involves changing your habits. You work to reshape your lifestyle by breaking unhealthy old habits that sabotage your weight and adopting healthy, new habits that will lead you down a path toward better health, including better heart health.

The Mayo Clinic Diet has two phases:

✔ Lose It! This two-week phase is designed to help you begin seeing weight-loss results right away.
✔ Live It! This second phase builds on Lose It! and is designed to help you continue to lose weight at a rate of 1 to 2 pounds a week until you reach your weight goal. This phase also helps you maintain your weight goal permanently by encouraging lifelong healthy habits.

Mediterranean diet

If you're looking for a heart-healthy eating plan, the Mediterranean diet might be right for you. The Mediterranean diet incorporates the basics of healthy eating — plus a splash of flavorful olive oil and perhaps a glass of red wine — in addition to other components that characterize the traditional cooking style of countries bordering the Mediterranean Sea. Research has shown that the traditional Mediterranean diet reduces the risk of heart disease.

The Mediterranean diet revolves around the following principles:
- ✔ Getting plenty of exercise
- ✔ Eating primarily plant-based foods, such as fruits and vegetables, whole grains, legumes, nuts and seeds
- ✔ Replacing butter with healthy fats, such as olive oil
- ✔ Using herbs and spices instead of salt to flavor foods
- ✔ Eating fish and poultry at least twice a week
- ✔ Drinking red wine in moderation (optional)

DASH diet

DASH stands for Dietary Approaches to Stop Hypertension. The DASH diet is a lifelong approach to healthy eating that's designed to help treat or prevent high blood pressure (hypertension). The diet encourages you to reduce the sodium in your diet and eat a variety of foods rich in nutrients that help lower blood pressure.

The DASH diet emphasizes:
- ✔ Limiting sodium to 2,300 milligrams a day (a modified version of the DASH diet sets sodium limits at 1,500 milligrams daily)
- ✔ Eating a diet emphasizing fruits, vegetables and whole grains
- ✔ Limiting red meat, sweets and added sugars
- ✔ Increasing intake of foods rich in potassium, magnesium and calcium

>> Obstacle

A meal without meat just doesn't seem like a meal to me. Plus I want to make sure I'm getting enough protein.

The fact is that most Americans get enough protein in their diets. Adults generally need 10 to 35 percent of their daily total calories to come from protein. You can get this from just 2 to 3 ounces of cooked lean meat, poultry or fish, ½ cup cooked dry beans or 2 tablespoons of peanut butter.

>> Strategies

Here are a few tips for maintaining a healthy diet with adequate lean protein.

+ Try easing into meatless meals. Consider going meatless one day each week. If you don't like the idea of a whole day without meat, start with a couple of meatless dinners each week. Plan meals that feature entrees you like that can be made without meat, such as a lasagna, soup or pasta salad.

+ When your meals include meat, don't overindulge. Choose lean cuts and avoid oversized portions. A serving of protein should be no more than 3 ounces — or about the size of a deck of cards — and should take up no more than one-fourth of your plate.

+ If you're concerned about protein, substitute the other protein-rich foods for meat in your favorite recipes. Beans and legumes are great in casseroles and salads. Vegetarian refried beans make a good substitute for meat in burritos and tacos. And tofu is the perfect addition to stir-fry dishes.

)) Obstacle
My family doesn't like to try new foods, and it's too much work to make two different meals.

Family support is important when you're trying to eat healthy, but don't let your family stop you from trying something new or exploring different ways of preparing favorite foods. When your family sees you enjoying a meal, your good habits may eventually rub off on them, too. People underestimate their ability to change their tastes. For example, when people first try skim or low-fat milk, they often say that it tastes like water. But after they stick with it for a while, most of these same people say that whole milk tastes too rich.

)) Strategies
Here are changes that may help both you and your family enjoy tastes in common and get on the same healthy track.

+ Take it slow. Don't try to overhaul your family's diet overnight. Make a few small changes at a time. Eventually, these small changes add up, and soon you'll all be following a healthier eating plan.

+ Offer a favorite dish that's prepared using a different cooking method. For example, instead of frying pork chops or chicken breasts, bake or grill them.

+ Involve your family in meal planning. Ask family members what they'd like to try that's different and healthy. If they can choose,

they might be more willing to experiment.

+ Keep more fruits and vegetables in the house, and keep fruit in a location where it's visible. When looking for a snack, make it easy to grab bananas, pears or grapes.

+ Remember that by preparing healthy options, you're laying a foundation of health for your family. While it may take some transition, the future benefits are worth it.

》 Obstacle

I'm not good at menu planning. I never have the right ingredients around the house to make a healthy meal.

It always helps if you plan ahead, but you can wing it and still eat well. Remember that healthy eating doesn't have to be complicated or involve hard-to-find ingredients. When you go to the grocery store, stock up on some of the basics. If you have on hand foods and ingredients such as the ones suggested below, you'll be able to prepare a good meal.

》 Strategies

Here are a few examples of good foods and ingredients to always have on hand.

+ Plenty of fruits and vegetables, including canned tomato products and vegetable soups and broth.

+ Lentils and beans, such as black beans, kidney beans and garbanzos.

+ Low-fat or fat-free milk, low-fat or fat-free cottage cheese, and reduced-fat cheeses.

+ Kitchen staples that you know you'll frequently use, such as salt and pepper. Add to your weekly shopping lists fresh produce, meat, dairy and bakery goods.

+ Skinless chicken and turkey, unbreaded fish, extra-lean ground beef, and round or sirloin beef cuts.

+ Cooking spray, olive oil and trans fat-free margarine.

+ Condiments, seasonings and spreads such as low-fat or fat-free salad dressings, herbs, spices, flavored vinegars, hummus and salsa.

+ Whole-grain breads, bagels and pita bread, low-fat tortillas, oatmeal, brown and white rice, whole-grain pasta, and whole-grain cereals that aren't pre-sweetened.

How to read a nutrition label

Keep these simple tips in mind:

❶ **Check the serving size.**
How many servings are in the container?

❷ **Check the calories in one serving.**

❸ **Check the % Daily Value.***
5 % or less is low
20 % or more is high

*Percent Daily Value (DV) in one serving is based on a 2,000-calorie diet for adults. For example, the recommended goal for dietary fiber is 25 grams, so 1 gram is 4% DV. Your DV may be higher or lower, depending on your calorie needs.

**Keep intake of saturated fat and trans fat as low as possible. All fats are high in calories.

Adapted from FDA, Center for Food Safety and Applied Nutrition, 2006

Nutrition Facts

❶ Serving Size 16 Crackers (31 g)
Servings Per Container About 9

❷ **Amount Per Serving**
Calories 150   Calories from Fat 50

❸   **% Daily Value***

Total Fat 6 g**	**9**%
Saturated Fat 1 g	**6**%
Trans Fat 1 g	
Polyunsaturated Fat 2 g	
Monounsaturated Fat 2 g	
Cholesterol 0 mg	**0**%
Sodium 270 mg	**11**%
Total Carbohydrate 21 g	**7**%
Dietary Fiber 1 g	**4**%
Sugars 3 g	
Protein 8 g	

Vitamin A 4%	Vitamin C 2%
Calcium 20%	Iron 4%

Limit nutrients shown in orange

Get enough of nutrients shown in green

)) Obstacle

Many of my favorite recipes are far from healthy, but I would rather not give them up.

Maybe it's your grandma's beloved bread pudding recipe, loaded with whole milk and eggs, or your own hit casserole smothered in cheese — delicious, but not exactly nutritious. But rather than throwing out that recipe card, first try making some ingredient or technique tweaks. You might be surprised at how close the new version tastes to the original.

)) Strategies

Here are five techniques you can use to transform your recipes into healthy ones.

+ Reduce the amount of fat, sugar and salt. You can do this without sacrificing flavor.

+ Make a healthy substitution. They not only reduce the fat, calories and salt in your recipes, but also boost nutrition. See the chart on the next page for substitution tips.

+ Cut back some ingredients. In some recipes, you can eliminate an ingredient altogether or scale back the amount you use. Eliminate items you add out of habit or for appearance, such as frosting, coconut or whipped toppings — all of which are high in fat and calories. Decrease condiments, such as pickles, olives, butter, mayonnaise, syrup, jelly,

mustard and soy sauce, which can have large amounts of salt, sugar, fat and calories.

+ Change cooking and prep techniques. Healthy cooking techniques — such as braising, broiling, grilling, poaching, sauteing and steaming — can capture the flavor and nutrients of your food without adding excessive fat or salt.

+ Downsize the portion size. No matter how many changes you try, some recipes may still be high in sugar, fat or salt. Try cutting back on the portion size instead.

Adapting recipes

If the recipe calls for	Try some of these substitutes
Butter **Margarine** **Shortening** **Oil**	<ul><li>For sandwiches, substitute tomato slices, ketchup or mustard.</li><li>For stovetop cooking, saute food in broth or small amounts of healthy oil like olive, canola or peanut or use cooking spray.</li><li>In marinades, substitute diluted fruit juice, wine or balsamic vinegar.</li><li>In cakes or bars, replace half the fat or oil with the same amount of applesauce, prune puree or commercial fat substitute.</li><li>To avoid dense, soggy or flat baked goods, don't substitute oil for butter or shortening, or substitute diet, whipped or tub-style margarine for regular margarine.</li></ul>
Meat	Keep it lean. In soup, chili or stir-fry, replace most of the meat with beans or vegetables. As an entree, keep meat to no more than the size of a deck of cards, and load up on vegetables.
Whole milk (regular or evaporated)	Use fat-free or 1% milk, or evaporated skim milk.
Whole egg (yolk and white)	Use ¼ cup egg substitute or 2 egg whites for breakfast or in baked goods.
Sour cream **Cream cheese**	Use fat-free, low-fat or light varieties in dips, spreads, salad dressings and toppings. Fat-free, low-fat and light varieties do not work well for baking.
Sugar	In most baked goods, you can reduce the amount of sugar by one-half without affecting texture or taste, but use no less than ¼ cup sugar for every cup of flour to keep items moist.
White flour	Replace half or more of white flour with whole-grain pastry or regular flour.

» Obstacle
I eat when I'm stressed, depressed or bored.

Sometimes your most intense longings for food happen right when you're at your weakest emotional points. Many people turn to food for comfort — be it consciously or unconsciously — when they're dealing with difficult problems or looking for something to distract their minds.

» Strategies
To help keep food out of your mood, try these suggestions.

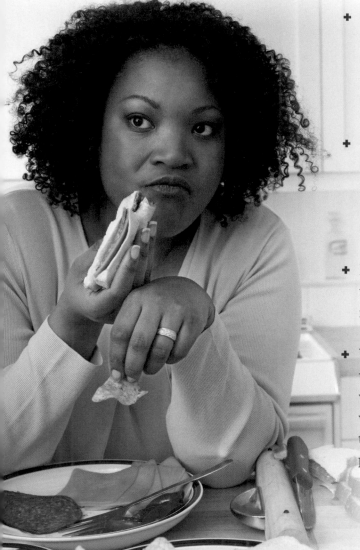

+ Try to distract yourself from eating by calling a friend, running an errand or going for a walk. When you can focus your mind on something else, the food cravings quickly go away.

+ Don't keep comfort foods in the house. If you turn to high-fat, high-calorie foods whenever you're upset or depressed, make an effort to get rid of them.

+ Identify your mood. Often the urge to eat can be attributed to a specific mood and not to physical hunger.

+ When you feel down, make an attempt to replace negative thoughts with positive ones. For example, write down all of the positive qualities about yourself and what you plan to achieve by getting healthy.

)) Obstacle
I have trouble controlling how much I eat.

For many people, a major struggle with how they eat is portion control. Part of the problem is they don't have a realistic idea of what constitutes a serving. In an era of jumbo meals, supersizing and free refills, overgenerous portions of food and beverages have become the norm. In addition, eating habits that you learned from a young age — that it's OK to have seconds, that you should clean your plate — can be difficult to break. But difficult doesn't mean impossible.

)) Strategies

You can train your body to feel full with less food, in the same way that your body became accustomed to needing more food to feel full. Try these suggestions.

+ Serve meals already dished onto plates instead of placing serving bowls on the table. This requires you to think twice before having a second portion.

+ Try using a smaller plate or bowl to make less food seem like more.

+ Eat slowly. When you eat too fast, your brain doesn't get the signal that you're full until after you've overeaten.

+ Eat foods that are healthy and low in calories first, before turning your attention to higher calorie foods.

+ Focus on your meal and on your company. Watching TV, reading or working often leads to mindless eating.

+ Stop eating as soon as you begin to feel full. You don't need to clean your plate.

+ Designate one area of the house to eat meals and only sit there when you eat.

+ If you're still hungry after finishing what's on your plate, nibble on a low-calorie food, such as fresh vegetables, fruit or crackers.

+ Portion sizes in restaurants can be two to three times the amount you need. Request a carryout container to take the excess home.

)) Obstacle
I've tried to make changes in my diet before but seem to never succeed at making them stick.

For many people, eating right and getting healthy can be a challenge. Don't be discouraged if you've tried changing how you eat in the past and you weren't able to — or if you relapsed.

)) Strategies
Following these tips may help you succeed this time around.

+ Change gradually. To boost your success, avoid dramatic changes in your eating approach. Instead, change one or two things at a time. If you now eat only one or two servings of fruit or vegetables a day, try to add a serving at lunch and one at dinner. Replace between-meal snacks with fruits and veggies.

+ Forgive yourself if you backslide. Everyone slips, especially when learning something new. Remember that changing your lifestyle is a long-term process. Find out what triggered your setback and then just pick up where you left off with your chosen diet.

+ Reward successes. Reward yourself with a nonfood treat — such as a new book or CD or a massage — for your accomplishments.

+ Add physical activity. To boost your heart-healthy efforts even more, consider increasing your physical activity in addition to following your new diet. Combining both a healthy diet and physical activity makes it more likely that you'll reduce your heart risks.

+ Get support if you need it. If you're having trouble keeping how you eat healthy, talk to your doctor or dietitian about it. You might get some tips that will help you stick to the eating plan.

10-minute (or less) meal ideas

Sauteed vegetables

Saute cherry tomatoes, asparagus, bell peppers, broccoli, onion and other vegetables. Toss with cooked whole-wheat pasta and a splash of olive oil. Top with grated Parmesan cheese.

Vegetables = multiple servings

1/2 cup pasta = 1 Carbohydrate

1 teaspoon oil = 1 Fat

Stir-fry

Cook quick brown rice while also stir-frying a bag of mixed, ready-to-eat vegetables in a little peanut oil. Toss vegetables with a teaspoon of Thai peanut sauce to spice up the flavor.

Vegetables = multiple servings

1/3 cup rice = 1 Carbohydrate

Use only a small amount of oil and sauce (1 teaspoon each) to count as 1 fat

Summer salad

Top bed of crisp romaine lettuce with a thinly sliced fresh (or canned in juice) whole pear. Sprinkle with four chopped pecans. Add a few shavings of Parmesan cheese. Drizzle with low-fat French dressing.

Lettuce = 1 Vegetable

Pear = 1 Fruit

Pecans & dressing = 2 Fat

(Parmesan not enough to count)

Quick soup

Bring to boil 1 quart reduced-sodium chicken broth. Cook any amount of fresh or leftover vegetables (for example, carrots, onions, green beans, mushrooms, rutabagas, tomatoes or zucchini) until vegetables are tender. Serve with 8 whole-wheat crackers or a slice of whole-wheat toast.

Vegetables = multiple servings

Crackers or toast = 1 Carbohydrate

Heart-healthy recipes

Grilled Asian salmon - SERVES 4

1 T sesame oil

1 T reduced-sodium soy sauce

1 T fresh minced ginger

1 T rice wine vinegar

4 4-oz. salmon fillets

PER SERVING

Calories	190
Total fat	11 g
Cholesterol	60 mg
Sodium	200 mg
Fiber	0 g

1. Combine sesame oil, soy sauce, ginger and vinegar in a shallow glass dish.
2. Add the salmon and turn to coat all sides. Refrigerate for 30 to 60 minutes, turning occasionally. Preheat the grill to medium-high heat.
3. Lightly oil the grill and place the salmon on the grill. Grill about 5 minutes a side. Fish is cooked when a knife blade inserted into the center reveals that the pink flesh is almost opaque. Serve warm.

Puttanesca with brown rice - SERVES 4

4 cups chopped ripe plum tomatoes

4 Kalamata olives, pitted and sliced

4 green olives, pitted and sliced

1½ T capers, rinsed and drained

1 T minced garlic

1 T olive oil

¼ cup chopped fresh basil

1 T fresh minced parsley

⅛ tsp. red pepper flakes

3 cups cooked brown rice

1. In a large bowl, combine the tomatoes, olives, capers, garlic and oil.
2. Add the basil, parsley and red pepper flakes, stirring to combine.
3. Cover and let stand at room temperature for 20 to 30 minutes, stirring occasionally.
4. Serve over the hot cooked rice.

PER SERVING

Calories	240
Total fat	7 g
Cholesterol	0 mg
Sodium	200 mg
Fiber	4 g

Chicken stir-fry with eggplant and basil - SERVES 4

¼ cup (⅓ oz.) coarsely chopped fresh basil

2 T chopped fresh mint

¾ cup (6 fl oz.) chicken stock or broth

3 green (spring) onions, including tender green
   tops, 2 coarsely chopped and 1 thinly sliced

2 cloves garlic

1 T peeled and chopped fresh ginger

2 T extra-virgin olive oil

1 small eggplant, with peel, diced (about 4
   cups)

1 yellow onion, coarsely chopped

1 red bell pepper, seeded and cut into julienne

1 yellow bell pepper, seeded and cut into
   julienne

1 lb skinless, boneless chicken breasts, cut into
   strips ½ inch wide and 2 inches long

2 T low-sodium soy sauce

PER SERVING

Calories	**248**
Total fat	**8 g**
Cholesterol	**66 mg**
Sodium	**408 mg**
Dietary fiber	**4 g**

1. In a blender or food processor, combine the basil, mint, ¼ cup of stock, chopped green onions, garlic, and ginger. Pulse until the mixture is minced but not puréed. Set aside.

2. In a large, nonstick frying pan, heat 1 tablespoon of olive oil over medium-high heat. Add eggplant, yellow onion, and bell peppers and sauté until the vegetables are just tender, about 8 minutes. Transfer to a bowl and cover with a kitchen towel to keep warm.

3. Add the remaining 1 tablespoon olive oil to the pan and heat over medium-high heat. Add the basil mixture and sauté for about 1 minute, stirring constantly. Add chicken strips and soy sauce and sauté until the chicken is almost opaque throughout, about 2 minutes.

4. Add the remaining ½ cup of stock and bring to a boil. Return eggplant mixture to the pan and stir until heated through, about 3 minutes. Transfer to a warmed serving dish and garnish with the sliced green onion. Serve immediately.

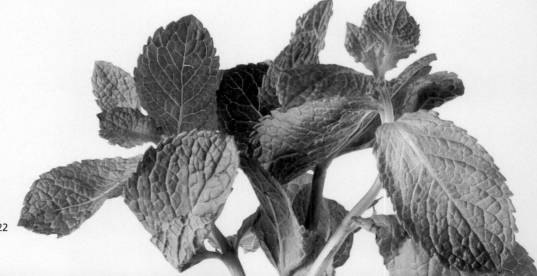

Grilled flank steak salad with roasted corn vinaigrette - SERVES 6

3 cups fresh corn kernels or frozen corn kernels, thawed

½ cup vegetable stock, no salt added

2 T fresh lime juice

2 T chopped red bell pepper

2 T extra-virgin olive oil

½ tsp. freshly ground black pepper

¼ cup chopped fresh cilantro (fresh coriander)

1 T ground cumin

2 tsp. dried oregano

¼ tsp. red pepper flakes

¾ lb. (12 oz.) flank steak

1 large head romaine lettuce, trimmed and torn into bite-sized pieces

4 cups cherry tomatoes, halved

¾ cup thinly sliced red onion

1½ cups cooked black beans, no salt added

1. Cook the corn in a large cast iron or heavy nonstick frying pan over medium-high heat, stirring often, until the corn begins to brown, 4 to 5 minutes, and then set aside.

2. In a food processor, combine stock, lime juice, bell pepper and 1 cup of roasted corn. Pulse to purée. Add olive oil, ¼ tsp. of black pepper and cilantro. Pulse to blend. Set the vinaigrette aside.

3. Preheat a grill or broiler. Away from the heat source, lightly coat a grill rack or broiler pan with cooking spray, and then position it 4 to 6 inches from the heat source.

4. In a small bowl, mix together cumin, oregano, red pepper flakes and ¼ tsp. black pepper. Rub on both sides of the steak. Grill or broil the steak, turning once, until browned, 4 to 5 minutes on each side. Cut into the center to check for doneness. Let stand for 5 minutes. Cut across the grain into thin slices. Cut the slices into pieces 2 inches long.

5. In a large bowl, combine lettuce, tomatoes, onion, black beans and remaining roasted corn. Add the vinaigrette and toss gently to mix well and coat evenly.

6. To serve, divide the salad among individual plates. Top each serving with slices of grilled steak..

PER SERVING

Calories	309
Total fat	7 g
Cholesterol	28 mg
Sodium	243 mg
Dietary fiber	10 g

Couscous salad - SERVES 8

1 cup whole-wheat Moroccan couscous*

1 cup zucchini, cut into ¼-inch pieces

1 medium red bell pepper, cut into ¼-inch pieces

½ cup finely chopped red onion

¾ tsp. ground cumin

½ tsp. ground black pepper

½ cup reduced-fat Italian dressing

Chopped fresh parsley or basil for garnish (optional)

PER SERVING

Calories	80
Total fat	1 g
Cholesterol	0 mg
Sodium	240 mg
Dietary fiber	2 g

1. *Follow preparation instructions on the package for cooking couscous. Instant couscous may be prepared by simply pouring boiling water over it, while traditional Moroccan couscous requires longer cooking.

2. When couscous is cooked, fluff with fork. Mix in zucchini, bell pepper, onion, cumin and black pepper. Pour Italian dressing over the mixture and toss to combine. Cover and refrigerate for 8 hours. Add garnish before serving.

Turkey veggie sloppy joes - SERVES 10

1 lb. ground turkey breast meat
    (or 12 oz. soy-based crumbles)

½ onion, finely chopped (about ¾ cup)

1 carrot, finely chopped

½ green bell pepper, chopped

1½ cups chopped zucchini squash

3 garlic cloves, minced

1 6-oz. can no-salt-added tomato paste

1½ cups water

1 T mild chili powder

1 tsp. paprika

1 tsp. dried oregano

½ tsp. ground black pepper

5 oz. reduced-fat cheddar cheese,
    thinly sliced

10 whole-wheat hamburger buns

1. In a large skillet over medium-high heat, sauté ground turkey until browned, about 7 minutes. Add onion and sauté 2 minutes. Add carrot and green pepper and sauté 2 minutes. Add zucchini and garlic and sauté 2 minutes more.

2. Add tomato paste and water, stirring until the paste has dissolved. Add chili powder, paprika, oregano and pepper. Reduce heat to medium and continue to cook until the mixture has thickened, about 10 minutes.

3. Preheat broiler. Divide cheese among the bottom halves of the hamburger buns. Transfer both halves of the buns to the broiler, open-faced, and toast until the cheese has melted and the buns are toasted.

4. Remove buns from the broiler and fill each sandwich with the meat-vegetable mixture. Serve immediately.

PER SERVING

Calories	230
Total fat	5 g
Cholesterol	35 mg
Sodium	340 mg
Dietary fiber	5 g

Minestrone soup - SERVES 4

1 T extra-virgin olive oil

½ cup chopped onion

⅓ cup chopped celery

1 carrot, diced

1 garlic clove, minced

4 cups fat-free, unsalted chicken broth

2 large tomatoes, seeded and chopped

½ cup chopped fresh spinach

1 (16-oz.) can chickpeas, no salt added

½ cup uncooked small-shell pasta

1 small zucchini, diced

2 T chopped fresh basil

1. In a large saucepan, heat the olive oil over medium heat.
2. Add the onion, celery and carrot and sauté until softened, about 5 minutes. Add garlic and continue cooking for another minute.
3. Stir in broth, tomatoes, spinach, chickpeas and pasta. Bring to a boil over high heat. Reduce heat and simmer for 10 minutes. Add zucchini. Cover and cook for 5 minutes more.
4. Remove from heat and stir in the basil. Ladle into individual bowls and serve immediately.

PER SERVING

Calories	190
Total fat	4 g
Cholesterol	5 mg
Sodium	215 mg
Dietary fiber	8 g

Springtime pea soup - SERVES 5

1 tsp. olive oil

3½ cups chicken broth, no salt added

1 medium onion, chopped

1 lb. frozen baby peas, thawed

2 medium potatoes, peeled and cut into ½-inch pieces

2 T reduced-fat sour cream

PER SERVING

Calories	140
Total fat	2 g
Cholesterol	5 mg
Sodium	100 mg
Dietary fiber	5 g

1. Heat the oil in a large pan over medium to high heat. Add onion and cook for about 2 minutes until the onion is softened.
2. Add the potato and cook, stirring, for about 2 more minutes. Add the chicken broth, cover and simmer for about 15 minutes, or until the potato is tender. Add peas and simmer for 5 minutes.
3. Purée in batches in a blender (use caution when blending hot liquids) until smooth. Reheat the soup. Ladle the soup into bowls and top with a dollop of sour cream.

Apple lettuce salad

15 MINUTES PREPARATION TIME ✚ SERVES 4

¼ cup unsweetened apple juice

2 tbsp. lemon juice

1 tbsp. canola oil

2¼ tsp. brown sugar

½ tsp. Dijon mustard

¼ tsp. apple pie spice

1 medium red apple, chopped

6 cups spring mix salad greens

1. Mix the apple juice, lemon juice, oil, brown sugar, apple pie spice and mustard in a large salad bowl.

2. Add the apple and toss to coat.

3. Add the salad greens and toss to mix just before serving.

PER SERVING

Calories	80
Total fat	4 g
Cholesterol	0 mg
Sodium	20 mg
Dietary fiber	3 g

Mixed berry whole-grain coffee cake - SERVES 8

½ cup skim milk

1 T vinegar

2 T canola oil

1 tsp. vanilla

1 egg

1/3 cup packed brown sugar

1 cup whole-wheat pastry flour

½ tsp. baking soda

½ tsp. ground cinnamon

1/8 tsp. salt

1 cup frozen mixed berries, such as blueberries, raspberries and blackberries (do not thaw)

¼ cup low-fat granola, slightly crushed

1. Heat oven to 350° F. Spray an 8-inch round cake pan with cooking spray and coat with flour.
2. In large bowl, mix the milk, vinegar, oil, vanilla, egg and brown sugar until smooth. Stir in flour, baking soda, cinnamon and salt just until moistened. Gently fold half the berries into the batter. Spoon into the prepared pan. Sprinkle with remaining berries and top with the granola.
3. Bake 25 to 30 minutes or until golden brown and top springs back when touched in center. Cool in pan on cooling rack 10 minutes. Serve warm.

PER SERVING

Calories	160
Total fat	5 g
Cholesterol	25 mg
Sodium	140 mg
Dietary fiber	3 g

Baked apples with cherries and almonds - SERVES 6

⅓ cup (1½ oz.) dried cherries, coarsely chopped

3 T chopped almonds

1 T wheat germ

1 T firmly packed brown sugar

½ tsp. ground cinnamon

⅛ tsp. ground nutmeg

6 small Golden Delicious apples, about 1¾ lb. total weight

½ cup (4 fl oz.) apple juice

¼ cup (2 fl oz. water

2 T dark honey

2 tsp. walnut oil or canola oil

PER SERVING

Calories	179
Total fat	4 g
Cholesterol	0 mg
Sodium	5 mg
Dietary fiber	5 g

1. Preheat the oven to 350°F.
2. In a small bowl, toss together the cherries, almonds, wheat germ, brown sugar, cinnamon, and nutmeg until all the ingredients are evenly distributed. Set aside.
3. The apples can be left unpeeled, if you like. To peel the apples in a decorative fashion, with a vegetable peeler or a sharp knife, remove the peel from each apple in a circular motion, skipping every other row so that rows of peel alternate with rows of apple flesh. Working from the stem end, core each apple, stopping I inch from the bottom.
4. Divide the cherry mixture evenly among the apples, pressing the mixture gently into each cavity.
5. Arrange the apples upright in a heavy ovenproof frying pan or small baking dish just large enough to hold them. Pour the apple juice and water into the pan. Drizzle the honey and oil evenly over the apples, and cover the pan snugly with aluminum foil. Bake until the apples are tender when pierced with a knife, 50–60 minutes.
6. Transfer the apples to individual plates and drizzle with the pan juices. Serve warm or at room temperature.

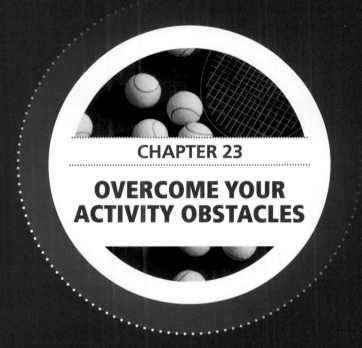

CHAPTER 23

OVERCOME YOUR ACTIVITY OBSTACLES

In Chapter 4 you learned how getting active — even in just small doses in a day — dramatically improves your heart health. But while you know exercise is important, starting and sticking with an exercise regimen or a more active lifestyle is often easier said than done.

That's where this chapter can help. Here, we've addressed some of the most common obstacles to physical activity and provided a number of practical tips to help you overcome them. Break down those barriers and get on your way to better health!

)) Obstacle
I don't have time to exercise.

Time for exercise is a common obstacle. With creativity and planning, you can overcome this obstacle. Perhaps you have more time than you realize. For example, the average American watches four hours of television each day. Add to that the time you may spend surfing the Web or going on minor errands in the car, and there's bound to be extra time for physical activity. In most cases, time really isn't the issue, rather it's a matter of priorities. To become more physically active, it may be that you need to give up another habit.

)) Strategies

If you can't find at least 30 minutes during your day to exercise, look for 10-minute windows. Exercising for 10 minutes three times a day is beneficial, too. Here are strategies you might try.

+ Remember that it's a heart boost to simply stand up and move around more in your day. Get up from your desk to stretch and walk around.

+ Walk for 10 minutes over your lunch hour, or get up a few minutes earlier in the morning and go for a short walk.

+ Take the stairs instead of the elevator, at least for a few floors.

+ Instead of always looking for the shortcut from one destination to another, look for opportunities to walk and get more physical activity in your day.

+ Develop a routine that you can do at home. While watching your favorite television program or reading, walk on a treadmill, ride a stationary bicycle or use an elliptical machine.

+ Use the community pool to swim laps or do water workouts.

+ Schedule time with a friend to do physical activities together on a regular basis.

+ While your child is at soccer practice or taking piano lessons, go for a walk or jog.

What's NEAT about physical activity

So your days are packed, or maybe you're just not a fan of dedicated exercise — that doesn't mean you can't get a good amount of activity into your daily routine. The answer for you might be to get NEAT.

NEAT stands for non-exercise activity thermogenesis, a concept pioneered by James A. Levine, M.D., an endocrinologist and researcher at Mayo Clinic. NEAT consists of all of the little movements that you perform during the day, such as tying your shoes, folding laundry and strolling over to the printer — energy expenditure that's not from purposeful exercise. Dr. Levine has found that increasing these types of activities will help you burn more calories and, therefore, lose weight and keep it off. And as noted in Chapter 4, these types of activities can also reduce your risk of heart disease by getting rid of sedentary time.

Little movements can add up in big ways. As Dr. Levine says, "If you simply convert sedentary TV time to active time, you could lose 50 pounds a year. Even marching in place or using a $50 stepper while watching your favorite programs would burn thousands of calories in a year and translate to a big weight loss."

Another great thing about increasing your NEAT activities throughout the day is that as you adapt to this more energized lifestyle, you will likely start to enjoy and pursue more vigorous types of physical activity. This will reduce your risk of heart disease even further.

See page 49 for examples of ways to increase your NEAT activities throughout your day.

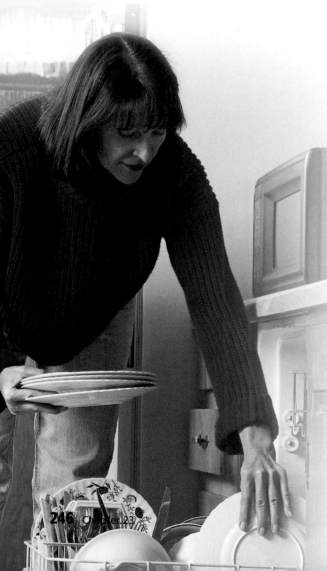

)) Obstacle

I don't like to exercise.

People who don't like to exercise generally view physical activity as painful or boring. It doesn't have to be either. From among the many forms of physical activity, you're bound to find something enjoyable. You need to experiment. Find something that piques your interest and try it out.

)) Strategies

Here are things you can do to help make exercise more enjoyable

+ Try not to focus on exercise only. Think of enjoyable things to do in which you're physically active, such as working in your flower garden or helping a friend with a house-building project. How you frame physical activity in your mind can make a big difference.

+ Take advantage of introductory classes or exercise videos to learn basic skills and techniques.

+ Mix things up. Don't feel tied to one activity, such as walking. On occasion, try biking or swimming instead.

+ Listen to music while you exercise. Upbeat music can rev you up and make your workout seem easier. It can also make the time pass more quickly.

+ Focus on the benefits of activity instead of the activity itself. Think of your workout time as personal time for you. Reflect on your goals and remind yourself how good it'll feel to achieve them.

+ Exercise with a friend or in a group. That way, you can socialize while you exercise, which may make the time go faster and the task seem less boring or painful.

)) Obstacle
I'm too tired to exercise.

Maybe that's because you're not exercising enough. Many people find they're less tired once they're involved with an exercise program. That's because regular physical activity gives you more energy and because fatigue is more often mental than it is physical. If you're fatigued due to stress, exercise is a great stress reliever.

)) Strategies
To incorporate more physical activity into your day, try these tips.

+ Begin with just five to 10 minutes of activity. Keep in mind that a little activity is better than none. And once you start, chances are you'll keep going for the full 10 minutes — if not longer.

+ Exercise in the morning. This will give you more energy throughout the day.

+ When you get home from work, don't sit down to watch television or use the computer. Instead, put on your walking shoes as soon as you arrive home and go for a walk.

+ Keep motivational messages where you need them to remind you of your goal.

)) Obstacle
I worry that other people will think I look funny when I exercise.

Try putting aside such thoughts. Most active people will give you credit for exercising and not make fun of you. Ask yourself which is more important: avoiding feeling possible embarrassment or getting healthy. Once you get started, you may find that exercising isn't as embarrassing as you thought it would be.

)) Strategies
If you're concerned about exercising in front of others, consider these suggestions.

+ Most of your self-consciousness will disappear as exercise becomes more routine and you become more confident.

+ Sign up for an exercise class that includes people at about the same age and fitness level as you.

+ Buy an exercise video or an exercise machine, such as a stationary bicycle or treadmill, so that you can work out in the privacy of your own home.

+ Exercise early in the morning or late in the evening, when fewer people are around.

+ Ask an exercise professional to demonstrate proper technique and provide information on appropriate exercises so that you can feel confident in your abilities.

)) Obstacle

It's too expensive to get in shape. I can't afford a gym membership or any of the fancy new equipment.

If the only thing keeping you from starting a fitness program is the cost of a gym membership, here's good news. You don't need to join a gym or buy pricey home equipment to take physical activity seriously. Plenty of low-cost alternatives can help you get fit.

)) Strategies

Here are a few ways to get in shape without breaking the bank.

+ Do strengthening exercises at home. Use inexpensive resistance bands — lengths of elastic tubing that come in varying strengths — in place of weights. Lift plastic milk jugs partially filled with water or sand. Do push-ups or squats using your body weight.

+ Watch an exercise video. Try videos on dance aerobics, cardio kickboxing, yoga or tai chi. For variety, trade exercise videos with a friend or check them out from the library.

+ Start a walking group. Round up friends, neighbors or co-workers for regular group walks. Plan routes through your neighborhood or near your workplace, along local parks and trails, or in a shopping mall.

+ Take the stairs. Skip the elevator when you can. Better yet, make climbing stairs a workout in itself.

+ Try your community center. Exercise classes offered through a local recreation department or community education group might fit your budget better than an annual gym membership.

+ Join in the fun. If you have children or grandchildren, don't just watch them play. Join them for a game of tag or kickball. Walk them to the park. Dance. Take a family bike ride or a group trip to the local pool.

>> Obstacle
I can't exercise because of painful arthritis in my joints.

For many people with chronic pain, exercise can be very beneficial. Physical activity can help you manage the symptoms of other chronic conditions. In the case of arthritis, proper exercise can help you maintain joint mobility.

>> Strategies

The key is knowing which exercises are helpful to your condition and which are harmful. If you have arthritis:

+ Try water exercises. The buoyancy of water takes the weight off your joints. You can swim laps on your own or you might try a water aerobics class.

+ Use a stationary or recumbent bicycle, which takes pressure off your knees.

+ Consider joining a basic yoga or tai chi class to increase strength and flexibility in your joints.

+ See a physical therapist who can offer recommendations on the best type of exercises for you. The therapist can also teach you how to do these exercises properly to avoid injury and further pain.

Exercise strategies for heart conditions

"There's been a major change in our thinking about exercise for people with heart disease," says Ray W. Squires, Ph.D., an exercise physiologist at Mayo Clinic. "If you go back 50 years, people were restricted to bed rest for weeks after a heart attack. Gradually we learned that was wrong."

People with heart disease and other heart-related problems need physical activity as much as anyone else. Even if you're not out playing football or running marathons, you can still reap numerous benefits from exercise. One of the best options is to participate in cardiac rehabilitation — also called cardiac rehab — a customized program of exercise and education designed to help you recover from a heart attack, other forms of heart disease, or heart surgery.

Cardiac rehabilitation is often divided into phases involving monitored exercise, nutritional counseling, emotional support and education about lifestyle changes that reduce your risks of future heart problems and increase your chance of survival. Cardiac rehabilitation is often covered by health insurance policies for many heart patients or may be available for a modest fee.

Even if you cannot participate in cardiac rehab, talk to your doctor about what activity is right for you. Something as simple as a regular walking program is a great place to start. Research shows that regular, brisk walking can reduce your risk of a heart attack. Other options to look into: yoga, tai chi, and even gentle water aerobics.

Keep it safe

To reduce the risk of injury while exercising, start slowly. Remember to warm up before you exercise and cool down afterward. Build up the intensity of your workouts gradually.

Stop exercising and seek immediate medical care if you experience any warning signs during exercise, including:

+ Chest pain or tightness
+ Dizziness or faintness
+ Pain in an arm or your jaw
+ Severe shortness of breath
+ An irregular heartbeat
+ Excessive fatigue

Know your limits — but achieve your potential

While it may seem slow going at first, many people with pre-existing conditions can work up to higher-intensity activity once they've gotten an OK from their doctor to do so. Dr. Squires thinks that many people with heart disease can benefit from higher intensity interval training when properly instructed and supervised — even older adults. As he notes, "We've had people who were in their 90s go through a program of interval training as a part of cardiac rehabilitation."

Be wise with weight training

Weight training can cause a temporary increase in blood pressure. This increase can be dramatic depending on how much weight you lift. But weight training can also have long-term benefits for blood pressure that outweigh the risk of a temporary spike for most people. If you have high blood pressure and want to include weight training in your fitness program, remember:

+ Use proper form when lifting to reduce the risk of injury. Don't hold your breath and avoid heavy straining. Doing so during exertion can cause dangerous spikes in blood pressure. Instead, breathe easily and continuously during each lift.

+ Lift lighter weights more times. Heavier weights require more strain, which can cause a greater increase in blood pressure. You can challenge your muscles with lighter weights by increasing the number of repetitions you do.

+ Listen to your body. Stop your activity right away if you become severely out of breath or dizzy or if you experience chest pain or pressure.

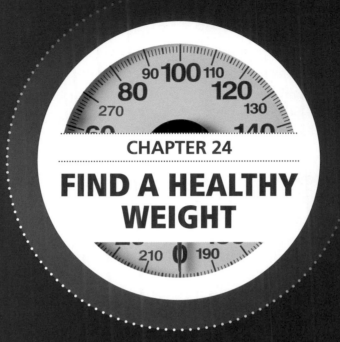

CHAPTER 24

FIND A HEALTHY WEIGHT

One of the best things you can do to keep your heart healthy is to be at a healthy weight. If you're obese, you're more likely to develop a number of serious health problems, including high cholesterol, high blood pressure and heart disease. But do you know what a healthy weight is for you? Or maybe you need some help getting there.

Simply put, a healthy weight means you have the right amount of body fat in relation to your overall body mass — but factors such as your height, age, sex, bone density and muscle mass, also may be taken into account.

You can also consider a healthy weight from another perspective. It's a weight that allows you to feel energetic, reduces your health risks, helps prevent premature aging (such as worn-out joints from carrying around too much weight) and improves your quality of life.

Stepping on the scale only tells you your total weight — including bone, muscle and fluid — but not how much of your weight is fat. The scale also doesn't tell you the locations on your body where you carry that fat. In determining your health risks, both of these factors are more important than is total weight.

So how do you know if you're at a healthy weight? While there are no objective standards for which weight "looks good," there are standards for what determines a healthy weight. The most common method is the National Institutes of Health approach based on three elements:

- ✔ Body mass index
- ✔ Waist measurement
- ✔ Medical history

Body mass index

Body mass index (BMI) is a tool for indicating your weight status. The mathematical calculation takes into account both your weight and height. BMI doesn't distinguish between fat and muscle but it more closely reflects the amount of body fat you have than does getting your weight measurement from a bathroom scale.

Although a BMI number is a good estimate of body fat for most people, it's not always a good match. Some people may have a high BMI but relatively little body fat.

For example, an athlete may be 6 feet 3 inches tall and weight 232 pounds, giving him a BMI of 29 — well above the classification of healthy weight. But he's not overweight because training has turned most of his weight into lean muscle mass.

By that same token, there may be some people who have a BMI in the healthy range but who carry a high percentage of body fat.

Waist measurement

Many conditions associated with being overweight or obese, such as high blood pressure, abnormal levels of blood fats, coronary artery disease, stroke, diabetes and certain types of cancer, are influenced by where the fat is located on your body.

Fat distribution can make your body look apple shaped or pear shaped. If you carry most of your fat around your waist or upper body, you're referred to as apple shaped. If most of your fat is around your hips and thighs or lower body, you're pear shaped.

When it comes to your health, it's better to have a pear shape than an apple shape. If you have an apple shape, you carry fat in and around your abdominal organs — which increases your risk of developing disease. If you have a pear shape, your risks aren't as high.

To determine whether you're carrying too much weight around your middle, measure your waist. Find the highest point on each hipbone and measure around your body just above those points. A measurement exceeding 40 inches in men or 35 inches in women indicates an apple shape and increased health risks.

Although these cutoffs of 40 and 35 inches are useful guides, there's nothing magic about them. It's enough to know that the bigger your waistline, the greater your health risks.

Medical history

Your BMI and waist measurement are essential numbers, but they don't give you the full picture of your weight status. A complete evaluation of your medical history also is important. In talking with your doctor about your weight, consider:

+ Do you have a family history of obesity, cardiovascular disease, diabetes, high blood pressure or sleep apnea? This may mean increased risk for you.

+ Have you gained considerable weight since high school? Even people with normal BMIs may be at

What's your BMI?

To determine your BMI, find your height in the left column. Follow that row across to the weight nearest yours. Look at the top of that column for your BMI number. Or use this formula:

1 Multiply your height (in inches) by your height (in inches) — or your height squared.
2 Divide your weight (in pounds) by the results of the first step.
3 Multiply that answer by 703. (For example, a 270-pound person, 68 inches tall, has a BMI of 41.)

	Normal		Overweight					Obese				
BMI	19	24	25	26	27	28	29	30	35	40	45	50
Height					Weight in pounds							
4'10"	91	115	119	124	129	134	138	143	167	191	215	239
4'11"	94	119	124	128	133	138	143	148	173	198	222	247
5'0"	97	123	128	133	138	143	148	153	179	204	230	255
5'1"	100	127	132	137	143	148	153	158	185	211	238	264
5'2"	104	131	136	142	147	153	158	164	191	218	246	273
5'3"	107	135	141	146	152	158	163	169	197	225	254	282
5'4"	110	140	145	151	157	163	169	174	204	232	262	291
5'5"	114	144	150	156	162	168	174	180	210	240	270	300
5'6"	118	148	155	161	167	173	179	186	216	247	278	309
5'7"	121	153	159	166	172	178	185	191	223	255	287	319
5'8"	125	158	164	171	177	184	190	197	230	262	295	328
5'9"	128	162	169	176	182	189	196	203	236	270	304	338
5'10"	132	167	174	181	188	195	202	209	243	278	313	348
5'11"	136	172	179	186	193	200	208	215	250	286	322	358
6'0"	140	177	184	191	199	206	213	221	258	294	331	368
6'1"	144	182	189	197	204	212	219	227	265	302	340	378
6'2"	148	186	194	202	210	218	225	233	272	311	350	389
6'3"	152	192	200	208	216	224	232	240	279	319	359	399
6'4"	156	197	205	213	221	230	238	246	287	328	369	410

Source: National Institutes of Health, 1998
*Asians with a BMI of 23 or higher may have an increased risk of health problems.

increased risk of weight-related conditions if they've gained more than 10 pounds since young adulthood.

+ Do you have a health condition, such as high blood pressure or type 2 diabetes, that would improve if you lost weight?

+ Do you smoke cigarettes or engage in little physical activity? These factors can compound the risk represented by excess weight.

Your BMI and waist measurement are snapshots of your current weight at the moment. The medical history helps reveal your risk of being overweight or of developing weight-related diseases over the long term.

So what's your ideal weight?

If your BMI shows that you're not overweight, if you're not carrying too much weight around your abdomen, and if you answered no to all of the medical history questions, there's probably little health advantage to changing your weight. (But you may still improve your health through a healthy diet and physical activity.)

If your BMI is between 25 and 29 or your waist measurement exceeds healthy guidelines, and you answered yes to one or more of the medical history questions, you'll probably benefit from losing a few pounds. Consult with your doctor before you start to lose weight.

If your BMI is 30 or more, you're considered obese. Losing weight should improve your health and reduce your risk of weight-related illnesses.

The Mayo Clinic Healthy Weight Pyramid

If you're looking for a fresh approach to weight loss, the Mayo Clinic Healthy Weight Pyramid is your answer.

The base of the pyramid focuses on generous amounts of food that contain a small number of calories in a large volume of food, particularly healthy fruits and vegetables. As the categories of the pyramid get narrower, you choose smaller amounts of food, including whole grains, lean protein and dairy, healthy fats, and even sweets.

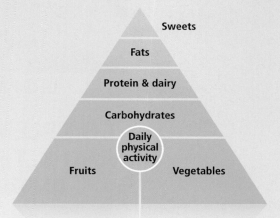

Fruits and vegetables. Fruits and vegetables are great sources of fiber, vitamins, minerals and other phytochemicals. They contain no cholesterol, are low in fat and sodium, and are high in essential minerals such as potassium and magnesium.

Carbohydrates. Carbohydrates, which are major energy sources for your body, include grain products, such as breads, cereals and pasta, and certain starchy vegetables such as potatoes and corn.

Protein and dairy. Foods rich in protein and relatively low in fat include beans and peas (legumes), fish, skinless poultry and lean meat. Low-fat or skim milk, yogurt and cheese have the same nutritional value as the whole-milk varieties but without the fat and calories.

Fats. As hard as it may be to believe, you need some fat in your diet. But not all fats are created equal. Look for liquid vegetable oils, such as olive or canola oils, rather than butter and margarine. But use all fats, including the healthier ones, sparingly.

Sweets. Foods in the sweets group are a high source of calories, mostly from sugar and fat. And they offer little in terms of nutrition. You don't have to give up these foods entirely. But be smart about your selections and portion sizes.

Daily physical activity. The Mayo Clinic Healthy Weight Pyramid is not just about food. At the center of the pyramid is a circle that recognizes the important role physical activity plays in health and weight loss.

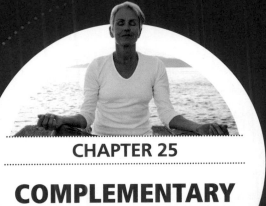

CHAPTER 25

COMPLEMENTARY AND ALTERNATIVE MEDICINE

Many people who are concerned about their health may turn to therapies that are not generally considered a part of conventional medicine. As many as 3 out of 4 Americans use complementary and alternative therapies such as yoga, acupuncture and dietary supplements. Among people with chronic conditions, including heart disease, or who have risk factors for heart disease, the percentage may even be higher.

Most people who use what's often considered nonconventional therapies also use conventional medicine. As a result, a term frequently used for alternative options is complementary and alternative medicine (CAM). CAM is sometimes called integrative medicine since it seeks to bring together (integrate) the best of both conventional medicine and nonconventional medicine.

An integrated approach to controlling heart disease may offer real benefits. A study at the Mayo Clinic found that a combination of diet, exercise and supplements, such as fish oil and red yeast rice, lowered cholesterol nearly as well as taking a prescription drug for lowering cholesterol. Mind-body approaches designed to relax the body and counteract the effects of stress also show promise in an integrated approach to managing high blood pressure — a risk factor for heart disease.

Many CAM therapies and approaches have been around for thousands of years. Others are newly discovered. However, until recently, there has been very little rigorous research of these therapies. This is changing as more researchers look into CAM options.

'Natural' does not mean 'safe'

Many people consider CAM therapies to be natural, and they equate natural with safe. Unfortunately, some CAM therapies carry risks and others just plain don't work. Even CAM therapies that offer possible benefits may also cause harmful interactions with other medications you're taking.

For example, the supplement St. John's wort, taken by some people for depression, can interfere with beta blockers, statins, blood thinners and other drugs. Even food-based supplements such as garlic, fish oil, saw palmetto and others can amplify the effects of aspirin and other blood thinners, leading to potentially dangerous bleeding situations.

Let your doctor know about all medications and herbal remedies you take — even those obtained without a prescription.

Common herbal and dietary supplements

Antioxidants: Coenzyme Q10 (CoQ10), vitamin C, vitamin E

Antioxidants are substances produced by the body and found in certain foods. They're also available as supplements. Some antioxidants are advertised as heart healthy, including CoQ10, vitamins C and E, and grape seed extract.

While there's evidence that a diet rich in antioxidants can be good for the heart, the same cannot be said for antioxidant supplements. For example, studies have provided little proof that taking vitamins C or E or beta carotene supplements can lower your risk of heart disease.

On the other hand, evidence suggests that CoQ10 may offer some heart benefits, such as lowering blood pressure or cholesterol. And having low levels of CoQ10 may be associated with a higher risk of heart failure.

But the news about CoQ10 isn't all good. CoQ10 may interact with prescription medications, including blood thinners. Check with your doctor first.

Oils: Omega-3 fatty acids, flaxseed

Omega-3 fatty acids help control inflammation, which plays an important role in heart health. However, the body does not make these essential ingredients itself. You can get them from food (including fish, flaxseed, walnut, canola and soy) but many people also take supplements.

Studies suggest omega-3 supplements may lower cholesterol and triglyceride levels, lower blood pressure, and reduce the risk of heart attack, stroke or death. The evidence is strongest for fish oil, but plant sources may also offer some benefits.

However, taking omega-3 supplements also carries some risk. Too much can increase the risk of bleeding and may affect the immune system. People scheduled for surgery should stop taking fish oil supplements three days before the procedure, if possible.

Herbs: Ginseng, hawthorn, ginkgo, garlic

For thousands of years, people have taken herbs for health reasons. In fact, many conventional medications come from herbs. Just as you wouldn't take medications without a prescription, you should consult a doctor before taking an herbal preparation.

Although there have been studies on the use of ginseng, hawthorn, ginkgo and garlic supplements to treat heart disease, there's little evidence that they're effective, and all of these herbal products may interfere with conventional heart medications.

Red yeast rice

Red yeast rice is not rice at all but an herb (also called hong qu). There's good evidence that it can lower total cholesterol, low-density lipoprotein (LDL) cholesterol and triglyceride levels. Under a doctor's supervision, it may offer an alternative to people who can't tolerate statins due to side effects.

Vitamin D

Vitamin D helps build healthy bones, but it may also play a role in heart health. Studies suggest that people with low levels of vitamin D may be more likely to have heart disease. Your doctor can easily check your vitamin D levels with a simple blood test. If you have a deficiency, your doctor may recommend taking a supplement.

Read the label

Before you buy or take a supplement, check the label for the following:

+ **Ingredients and dose:** Choose supplements that provide about 100 percent of the Daily Value (DV) of the vitamin or mineral, rather than a megadose of 500 percent of the DV. Ask your doctor how much you should take.

+ **USP certification:** USP stands for U.S. Pharmacopeia, a nonprofit organization that tests supplements to ensure they contain what the manufacturer claims.

+ **Expiration date:** Supplements can lose potency over time; discard once expired. If there is no date on a bottle, don't buy it.

Supplements should be stored in a dry, cool place, preferably a locked cabinet where children or pets cannot get to them. The National Center for Complementary and Alternative Medicine (nccam.nih.gov) and the Office of Dietary Supplements (ods.od.nih.gov) offer more information on supplement safety.

Food as medicine

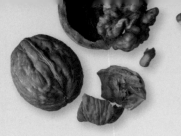

Diet is an important factor in heart health. The choices you make at mealtime — and in between — can make the difference between heart health and heart disease. According to one study, changing your diet can reduce your risk of heart disease by 60 percent. Add other lifestyle changes — such as regular exercise and stress management — and your risk may drop as much as 82 percent.

Vegetables and fruits are so important to heart health that they're a cornerstone of the Mayo Clinic Healthy Heart Plan. Studies consistently demonstrate their positive effect. Other kinds of food can also provide heart benefits:

Fish: Fish, especially salmon, tuna and herring, provides a good source of omega-3 fatty acids, which help lower blood pressure as well as cholesterol and triglyceride levels. Choose fish twice a week and prepare it by baking or broiling — frying eliminates the benefits.

Olive oil and polyunsaturated fats: Instead of reaching for butter, use polyunsaturated and monounsaturated fats that fight inflammation. Olive oil, which is high in monounsaturated fats, is great for cooking as well as a substitute for butter on bread. Look for virgin oil, which is minimally processed and preserves the micronutrients that add to its health benefits. Peanut, canola and flaxseed oils also are high in monounsaturated fats. Good choices of polyunsaturated fats include safflower, sunflower and nut oils.

Foods with added plant sterols or stanols: Foods are now available that have been fortified with sterols or stanols — substances found in plants that help block the absorption of cholesterol. Margarines, orange juice and yogurt drinks with added plant sterols can help reduce LDL cholesterol by more than 10 percent.

Cranberries: Cranberries — and cranberry juice — contain antioxidants. One study found that daily double-strength cranberry juice (54 percent juice) reduced arterial stiffness that's associated with atherosclerosis. However, cranberry juice may interact with blood thinners. Consult your doctor before increasing cranberry juice consumption.

Grapes (including wine): Grapes, grape juice and wine are excellent sources of antioxidants, which have been shown to lower LDL cholesterol levels. Some antioxidants may also reduce blood pressure, fight clotting and regulate heart rate. The darker the grape, the higher the antioxidant concentration in the fruit. However, too much fruit sugar and alcohol can undo the health benefits you gain. Talk to your doctor about a safe amount of alcohol to drink.

Dark chocolate and cocoa: Chocolate and cocoa contain high levels of antioxidant flavonoids, which can help lower blood pressure, lower cholesterol, and prevent inflammation and excessive clotting. These flavonoids may reduce the risk of death from heart disease.

Unfortunately, the most popular type of chocolate — milk chocolate — is high in saturated fat and sugar and low in cocoa. Dark chocolate, with higher amounts of flavonoids and less sugar and fat, has more potential. Some researchers recommend as much as 100 grams (about 3½ ounces) of dark chocolate a day for its heart benefits. Make sure that adding chocolate to your diet does not come at the cost of weight gain.

Tea and coffee: Tea and coffee also contain high amounts of flavonoids. One study found that people who drink tea and coffee are less likely to die of heart disease than those who don't. Tea appears to offer more protection than coffee: People who drank three to six cups of tea a day had a 45 percent lower risk of heart disease than those who drank less than a cup. For coffee, two to four cups a day lowered heart disease risk by 20 percent. Drink it black or use skim milk and don't add sugar.

Soybeans and other beans: Soybeans and other beans contain high amounts of fiber and antioxidants, both of which have heart benefits. Eating high amounts of soy appears to be an important dietary contributor to heart health. The benefit may come not only from the ingredients in soy and other beans but also from using beans to replace meat, especially high-fat red meat.

Nuts: Nuts, especially walnuts, almonds and pecans, contain heart-healthy unsaturated fats and help lower cholesterol. However, nuts are also full of calories. To get the benefits, but not the weight gain, eat no more than 1 to 3 ounces a day.

"Sticky" grains: Certain grains — especially oats and barley — contain soluble fiber, which reduces LDL cholesterol. Adding foods such as oatmeal or oat bran to your diet may help lower cholesterol significantly.

Mind-body medicine

Stress prompts your body to release hormones that raise blood pressure, speed up breathing and narrow blood vessels. This response pushes energy to the muscles and heart so that you're ready to take action against danger. But chronic stress damages the heart.

It makes sense, then, that the opposite of stress — relaxation — can help the heart. That's the basis for the use of mind-body medicine in preventing and treating heart disease.

Studies show that relaxation techniques may lower blood pressure, decrease lipid levels and increase a feeling of well-being that enhances your health overall. When combined with other lifestyle changes and conventional medical care, relaxation techniques may also reduce the risk of another heart attack.

Fit these mind-body methods into your day to bring on the relaxation response. You can easily learn and perform them on your own, although tapes, classes or other instruction is available. Regular practice of these techniques is a safe way to do your heart — and your head — some good.

Biofeedback

Unlike the other mind-body techniques discussed in this section, biofeedback typically requires a clinician and special equipment to decrease your stress response and increase your relaxation response. In biofeedback, the clinician attaches sensors to pick up your heart rate, blood pressure and body temperature. With this feedback, the clinician can guide you through methods of recognizing stress and making positive physical changes that cause relaxation. Through training, you can learn to control stress responses and bring on relaxation more easily.

If you have 5 minutes...

Listen to music. Studies show that listening to music may lower blood pressure and heart rate in people with heart disease. It also reduces anxiety in people recovering from heart attack. Classical music is more apt to calm you down than crank you up.

For another option, try progressive relaxation. Lie down in a comfortable position and focus on each muscle group, starting at your head and moving toward your toes. First tense, then release each muscle group while breathing slowly and thinking pleasant thoughts. Studies show that this technique can help lower blood pressure.

If you have 15 minutes...

Try meditation. Many people who meditate regularly report that it lowers anxiety and depression, both of which play a role in heart disease. While some people meditate for much longer periods of time, even 15 minutes can quiet the mind and refresh the spirit.

Types of meditation include mindfulness meditation, transcendental meditation, paced-breathing meditation and visualization. There are books and tapes that can teach you how to focus on your breathing or a mantra and keep an open attitude toward distractions. Some people prefer starting with a class, then practicing on their own.

If you have 60 minutes...

Join a tai chi, yoga or qi gong class or group. More and more community centers, gyms, and even workplace wellness programs offer classes and instruction in these ancient Asian arts.

Studies show that these techniques, which gracefully combine meditation and movement, may lower blood pressure, increase lung capacity, bring on relaxation and improve mood. Once you're familiar with the postures and movements of these arts, you can do the exercises on your own. But it may be best to start with a class, which usually lasts about an hour.

Acupuncture

Acupuncture, which involves the insertion of very thin needles to specific points and depths on the body, originated in China thousands of years ago. This ancient approach to medicine may hold promise in dealing with one of the most common ailments of the 21st century — heart disease. When added to conventional treatment, acupuncture may increase the ability of people who have heart failure to exercise. Some studies have shown that acupuncture may reduce blood pressure — and it may add to the effectiveness of blood pressure medication. More study is needed to learn more about this possible benefit.

CHAPTER 26

MONITOR YOUR MENTAL HEALTH

Stress, depression, anxiety — you might wonder what they have to do with your heart. The fact is that your mood can affect your long-term heart health, making it more likely for things to go wrong. Also, people who have a heart condition or have had a heart attack are more likely to experience depression or anxiety, which takes a further toll on your health.

Stress and your heart

Stress is a normal reaction to the demands of your life. Your brain comes hard-wired with an alarm system for your protection. When your brain perceives something that could be a threat, it signals the release of a burst of hormones that fuels your capacity to respond — the so-called fight-or-flight response. You quickly decide either to confront the threat or to avoid it.

Once the threat is gone, your body is meant to return to a normal relaxed state. Unfortunately, if there's nonstop stress in your life, your alarm system rarely shuts off.

By not staying in control of your stress level, your body is left on high alert. And over time, high levels of stress can lead to serious health problems.

You may respond to stress in ways that increase your risk of heart disease, high blood pressure or heart attack. For example, if you're under stress, you may overeat or smoke from nervous tension.

Or you may let healthy behaviors such as regular physical activity slide.

That's why managing your response to stress is important. Stress management provides you with a range of tools to help reset your alarm system. And by adopting healthy techniques for doing so, you'll help keep your mind and body in their best possible shape for years to come.

Managing your stress

If you can think of stress as your reaction to an event, rather than the event itself, it becomes easier to find ways of managing stress. You may not be able to control all of the causes, but you can control your response to them.

Look at your life and consider different stressors that you face every day. Divide them into four basic categories: things you can or can't control and things that are or are not important.

Create a chart similar to the one pictured below. Assign a few things that bother you to one of the four boxes, according to how well you think you can control them and how important you think they are.

Once you've assigned your stressors to the chart, consider different strategies for how to respond to them.

The more stressors you have in the box at upper left, the better it may be for you — those are important stressors that you can control or change.

Stressors in the box at upper right may be more perplexing. For some of them, you may need to learn acceptance and give up some of the anger and resentment you're feeling.

For stressors in the lower half of the chart, recognize when it may be best to "let go" — maybe you don't need to waste so much time and energy dealing with them.

	Can control	Can't control
Important	- Healthy eating, being physically active	- Relatives' behavior at family get-togethers
Less important	- Weeds in my garden	- Traffic congestion

Finding inner peace to relieve daily stress

"When some people hear the word 'meditation,' they worry that they'll have to sit in a lotus position for an hour and chant. But you can achieve the calming effects of meditation — and relieve stress — without formal, ritualized practice," says Amit Sood, M.D., Mayo Clinic.

"Traditional meditation models are good for people who are in a monastery, where they may not have as many stressors," he says. But for people who haven't practiced meditation, jumping right in can be like learning to drive on a busy highway. First, it's important to strengthen the ability to focus your attention. Here are three simple ways to start practicing relaxation:

1. **Start your morning in the here and now.** Most people start worrying within seconds of waking up. Begin your day in a more relaxed manner — which sets the tone for the rest of the day — by focusing on details around you. Pay attention to the feeling of your feet touching the carpet. Count the number of steps to the bathroom. Pause to enjoy the fragrance of soap and water. Focus on a here and now mode instead of a what-if mode.

2. **Spend 10 to 15 minutes a day with nature.** The soothing sounds, smells and sights of trees, grass, birds, flowers and wind can help counterbalance the eight hours you spend in front of a computer screen. "Nature does not ask anything of us," says Dr. Sood. "It is what it is."

3. **Transition mindfully from work to home.** Like in the morning, your transition from daytime to evening is critical. If you're coming from work, use the drive home to focus your attention on novel details around you, from the cars in the parking lot to the billboard signs to the clouds in the sky. Instead of taking your family for granted, greet them as if you haven't seen them for a long time.

Depression after a heart event

Depression is common after you've experienced a heart attack or undergone heart surgery or another heart-related procedure. You may feel that you can no longer do things you used to do — that you're not the same person you were before the event. It may be coupled with feelings of fear, anger and guilt.

Openly discussing these feelings with your doctor, a family member or a friend may help you better cope. You need to take care of yourself mentally as well as physically. Exercising and participating in cardiac rehabilitation sessions with other people in recovery may help you work through these feelings.

Linking depression and anxiety to heart health

Many people think of depression and anxiety as issues that are restricted to your mind. While it's true that these disorders influence your thoughts, moods, feelings and behaviors, your physical health is affected as well.

Depression and anxiety disorders may cause abnormal heart rhythms, higher blood pressure, and faster blood clotting, and lead to higher levels of insulin and cholesterol.

Chronic depression and anxiety may also result in elevated levels of stress hormones, which trigger the fight-or-flight response. Long term, this can increase your heart's workload and prevent your body from repairing tissue damaged by heart disease.

Depression can keep you from taking care of your health, which can increase your risk of heart disease. Persistent feelings of sadness, loss of interest in your usual activities and low self-esteem often lead to unhealthy lifestyle choices, such as eating a poor diet, engaging in little or no exercise, and abusing drugs and alcohol.

In addition, depression's impact on your mood and behaviors may make it harder to take medications or follow a treatment plan for heart disease or other conditions, such as high blood pressure or diabetes — which may lead to or worsen heart problems.

Recognizing depression

Depression is a medical illness that involves the mind and the body. Also called major depression, major depressive disorder and clinical depression, it affects how you feel, think and behave.

Depression can lead to many emotional and physical problems. You may have trouble doing normal day-to-day activities. Depression may make you feel as if life isn't worth living. Depression signs and symptoms include:

- Feelings of sadness or unhappiness
- Loss of interest or pleasure in normal activities
- Irritability or frustration, even over small matters
- Reduced sex drive
- Insomnia or excessive sleeping
- Changes in appetite — depression often causes decreased appetite and weight loss, but in some people it causes increased cravings for food and weight gain
- Agitation or restlessness — for example, pacing, hand-wringing or an inability to sit still
- Slowed thinking, speaking or body movements
- Indecisiveness, distractibility and decreased concentration
- Fatigue, tiredness and loss of energy — even small tasks seem to require a lot of effort
- Feelings of worthlessness or guilt, fixating on past failures or blaming yourself when things aren't going right
- Trouble thinking, remembering and making decisions
- Frequent thoughts of death, dying or suicide
- Crying spells for no apparent reason
- Unexplained physical problems, such as back pain or headaches

More than just a bout of the blues, depression isn't a weakness, nor is it something that you simply "snap out of." Depression is a chronic illness that often requires long-term management.

The good news is that effective treatments, such as medications and psychological counseling (psychotherapy), are available. Talk to your doctor for an assessment of your symptoms, especially if they're taking a toll on your life.

Self-care tips

Depression often does require professional treatment. The self-care strategies you can undertake are active, effective ways of managing depression, both on their own or combined with medication and therapy.

+ Get exercise. Numerous studies have found that physical activity reduces symptoms of depression. Consider walking, jogging, swimming, gardening or taking up any activity you enjoy.

+ Stick to your treatment plan. Don't skip therapy sessions or appointments, even if you don't feel like going. Talk to your doctor if you don't think a medication is helping or if you're bothered by side effects — changing the dose or the drug itself may help. Even if you're feeling well, resist any temptation to skip your medications. If you stop, depression symptoms may

▶ **De-stressing your life**
See Chapter 12 for other tips for helping you reduce your stress load and adapt to changes in your life.

come back, and you could also experience withdrawal-like symptoms.

+ Learn about depression. Education about your condition can empower and motivate you to stick to your treatment plan.

+ Watch the signs. Work with your doctor or therapist to learn what might trigger your symptoms. Contact a professional if you notice changes in symptoms or how you feel. Ask family members or friends to help watch for warning signs.

+ Avoid alcohol and drugs. In the long run, they generally make symptoms worse and make depression harder to treat.

+ Get plenty of sleep. Sleeping well is especially important when you're depressed. If you're having trouble sleeping, talk to your doctor.

Taking care of anxiety

Anxiety is a normal part of life. It can even be useful when it alerts us to danger. But for some people, anxiety is a persistent problem that interferes with daily activities. This type of anxiety can disrupt relationships and enjoyment of life, and over time it can lead to health concerns.

Common anxiety symptoms include:

- Constant worrying or obsession about small or large concerns
- Restlessness and feeling keyed up or on edge
- Difficulty concentrating
- Irritability
- Muscle tension or muscle aches
- Trembling, feeling twitchy or being easily startled
- Trouble sleeping
- Sweating, nausea or diarrhea
- Shortness of breath or a rapid heartbeat
- Avoidance of activities out of worry

The two main treatments for anxiety disorders are medications and psychotherapy. You may benefit most from a combination of the two.

Self-care tips

Apart from or in addition to professional treatment, lifestyle changes can make a big difference. Here are a few everyday steps that have shown to help keep anxiety under control.

+ Get exercise. Exercise is a powerful stress reducer. It's best if you develop a regular routine and work out most days of the week. Start out slowly and gradually increase the amount and intensity of the exercise you do.

+ Avoid alcohol and other sedatives. These can worsen anxiety.

+ Use relaxation techniques. Visualization, meditation and yoga are examples of relaxation techniques that can ease anxiety.

+ Make sleep a priority. Do what you can to make sure you're getting enough quality sleep. If you aren't sleeping well, see your doctor.

+ Quit smoking and cut back or quit drinking coffee. Both nicotine and caffeine can worsen anxiety.

MAYO CLINIC

HOUSECALL

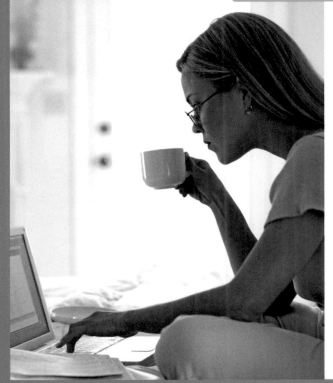

What our readers are saying ...

*"I depend on **Mayo Clinic Housecall** more than any other medical info that shows up on my computer. Thank you so very much."*

"Excellent newsletter. I always find something interesting to read and learn something new."

*"**Housecall** is a must read – keep up the good work!"*

*"I love **Housecall**. It is one of the most useful, trusted and beneficial things that come from the Internet."*

*"The **Housecall** is timely, interesting and invaluable in its information. Thanks much to Mayo Clinic for this resource!"*

"I enjoy getting the weekly newsletters. They provide me with friendly reminders, as well as information/conditions I was not aware of."

Get the latest health information direct from Mayo Clinic ... Sign up today, it's FREE!

Mayo Clinic Housecall is a FREE weekly e-newsletter that offers the latest health information from the experts at Mayo Clinic. Stay up to date on topics that are current, interesting, and most of all important to your health and the health of your family.

What you get
- Weekly featured topics
- Answers from the experts
- Quick access to our Symptom Checker
- Healthy recipes with nutritional values listed
- Videos and slide shows
- Health tip of the week
- And much more!

Don't wait ... Join today!
MayoClinic.com/Housecall/Register

We're committed to helping you enjoy better health and get the most out of life every day. We hope you decide to become part of the Mayo Clinic family, where you can always count on receiving an interesting mix of health information from a trusted source.

Image credits

NAME: DV1356052_22.PSD/PAGE: III/CREDIT: DIGITAL VISION/COLLECTION: DIGITAL VISION – NAME: © MAYO FOUNDATION FOR MEDICAL EDUCATION AND RESEARCH. ALL RIGHTS RESERVED – NAME: FAN2016322.PSD/PAGE: V - V/CREDIT: GETTY - NAME: 70104.PSD/PAGE: 8/CREDIT: PHOTODISC/COLLECTION: PHOTODISC – NAME: 75186.PSD/PAGE: 13/CREDIT: MICHAEL MATISSE/COLLECTION: PHOTODISC – NAME: FAN9003024.PSD/PAGE: 16/CREDIT: © MONALYN GRACIA/CORBIS/COLLECTION: CORBIS – NAME: FAN1006959-2.PSD/PAGE: 18/CREDIT: © GETTY/COLLECTION: GETTY – NAME: 22588AL-SRGB75.PSD/PAGE: 19/CREDIT: © STOCKBYTE/COLLECTION: STK – NAME: E000049R.PSD/PAGE: 21/CREDIT: © STOCKBYTE/COLLECTION: STK – NAME: WEE_029R.PSD/PAGE: 24/CREDIT: © EYEWIRE/COLLECTION: EYEWIRE – NAME: PAF090C0043-2.PSD/PAGE: 25/CREDIT: © EYEWIRE/COLLECTION: EYEWIRE – NAME: OS31085.PSD/PAGE: 26/CREDIT: © PHOTODISC/COLLECTION: PHOTODISC – NAME: 327083RKNRGB75.PSD/PAGE: 28/CREDIT: © STOCKBYTE/COLLECTION: STOCKBYTE – NAME: FAN9003079.PSD/PAGE: 31/CREDIT: © MONALYN GRACIA/CORBIS/COLLECTION: CORBIS - NAME: NAME: PAF089000004.PSD/PAGE: 36/COLLECTION: PHOTOALTO – NAME: PAF0E9000004.PSD/PAGE: 36/CREDIT: © EYEWIRE/COLLECTION: EYEWIRE – NAME: MSS_863767.PSD/PAGE: 39/CREDIT: © MFMER – NAME: PAF0E0000049.PSD/PAGE: 37/CREDIT: © ISABELLE ROZENBAUM/COLLECTION: PHOTOALTO – NAME: BXP49850H.PSD/PAGE: 39/CREDIT: © BRAND_X PICTURES COLLECTION/COLLECTION: BRAND_X PICTURES – NAME: AA050708.PSD/PAGE: 44/CREDIT: © TIM HALL/COLLECTION: DIGITAL VISION_8233.PSD/PAGE:45/CREDIT: © JULES FRAZIER/COLLECTION: PHOTODISC –NAME: MYPLATE_WHITE.PSD/PAGE: 45/CREDIT: © USDA – NAME: OS25006.PSD/PAGE: 45/CREDIT: © C SQUARED STUDIOS/COLLECTION: PHOTODISC – NAME: OS25058.PSD/PAGE: 45/CREDIT: © C SQUARED STUDIOS/COLLECTION: PHOTODISC – NAME: OS25092.PSD/PAGE: 45/CREDIT: © C SQUARED STUDIOS/COLLECTION: PHOTODISC – NAME: PYRAMID. PSD/PAGE: 45/CREDIT: © MFMER – NAME: OS28114.PSD/PAGE: 46/CREDIT: © C SQUARED STUDIOS/PHOTODISC/COLLECTION: PHOTODISC – NAME: BS25091.JPG/PAGE: 46/CREDIT: © SIEDE PREIS – NAME: SEN_003-2.PSD/PAGE: 46_47/CREDIT: © EYEWIRE COLLECTION/COLLECTION: PHOTODISC – NAME: 62985CORCMYK75.PSD/PAGE: 49/CREDIT: © STOCKBYTE ROYALTY FREE PHOTOS/COLLECTION: STOCKBYTE – NAME: FAN9003019.PSD/PAGE: 51/CREDIT: © MONALYN GRACIA/CORBIS – NAME: 00075321.PSD/PAGE: 54/CREDIT: © COMSTOCK/COLLECTION: COMSTOCK – NAME: 70183.PSD/PAGE: 53/CREDIT: © RYAN MCVAY/COLLECTION PHOTODISC – NAME: MSS_762420.PSD/PAGE: 50/CREDIT: © MFMER – NAME: 77097.JPG/PAGE: 56/CREDIT: © JULES FRAZIER/COLLECTION PHOTOD SC – NAME: 24086.PSD/PAGE 56_57/CREDIT: © STEVE COLE/GETTY IMAGES/COLLECTION: PHOTODISC – NAME: SS47056.PSD/PAGE: 58/CREDIT: © NICK KOUDIS/COLLECTION: PHOTODISC – NAME: 110079.PSD/PAGE: 59/CREDIT: © JANIS CHRISTIE/COLLECTION: PHOTODISC – NAME: OS48045BLUE.PSD/PAGE: 36, 50, 60, 67, 69, 86, 92, 109, 118, 151, 161, 172, 174, 181, 183, 191, 193, 203/CREDIT: © SIEDE PREIS/COLLECTION: PHOTODISC – NAME: MSS_517976.PSD/PAGE: 60/CREDIT: © MFMER – NAME: 327023RKNRGB75.PSD/PAGE: 61/CREDIT: © G2-12-15-04-LSL – NAME: 110075.PSD/PAGE: 63/CREDIT: © NANCY R. COHEN/COLLECTION: PHOTODISC – NAME: 67008.JPG/PAGE: 64/CREDIT: © DUNCAN SMITH/COLLECTION: PHOTODISC – NAME: SS36074.PSD/PAGE: 65/CREDIT: © THOMAS BRUMMETT/COLLECTION: PHOTODISC – NAME: HURT.PSD/PAGE: 67/ © MFMER – NAME: HENSRUD.PSD/PAGE: 69/ © MFMER – NAME: 42161.PSD/PAGE: 70/CREDIT: © JACK HOLLINGSWORTH/COLLECTION: PHOTODISC – NAME: 1040PENCILPATH.PSD/PAGE: 72/CREDIT: © PHOTOLINK/COLLECTION: PHOTOLINK – NAME: PAPERSCANYELLOW.JPEG/PAGE: 72/ © MFMER – NAME: 342130B.PSD/PAGE: 73/CREDIT: © DIGITAL VISION/COLLECTION: PHOTO_LINK – NAME: OS48057.PSD/PAGE: 75/CREDIT: © SIEDE PREIS/COLLECTION PHOTOLINK – NAME: THORNG.PSD/PAGE: 76/CREDIT: © MFMER – NAME: FERNANDEZ-2011_20.PSD/PAGE: 79/ © MFMER – NAME: OS38005PATH.PSD/PAGE: 82/CREDIT: © SIEDE PREIS/COLLECTION PHOTOLINK – NAME: TESTGREEN.PSD/PAGE: 82/CREDIT: © SIEDE PREIS/COLLECTION: PHOTOLINK –NAME: 565287C0.PSD/PAGE: 83/CREDIT: © GETTY IMAGES/STOCKBYTE/COLLECTION: STOCKBYTE – NAME: ACKERMAN.PSD/PAGE: 86/ © MFMER – NAME: TIPTON-HUBER.PSD/PAGE: 89/ © MFMER – NAME: OS25045.PSD/PAGE: 90/CREDIT: © C SQUARED STUDIOS/COLLECTION: C SQUARED STUDIOS - NAME: FAN1006999.PSD/PAGE: 91/CREDIT: © MFMER – NAME: RANDALTHOMAS.PSD/PAGE: 92/CREDIT: © MFMER – NAME: 496069. PSD/PAGE: 93/CREDIT: © DIGITAL VISION/COLLECTION: PHOTODISC – NAME: FAN9003030.PSD/PAGE: 97/CREDIT: © MONALYN GRACIA/CORBIS – NAME: 116086.PSD/PAGE: 98, 99/CREDIT: © AMOS MORGAN – NAME: SKD284342SDC_22.PSD/PAGE: 98/CREDIT: © GETTY IMAGES/STOCKDISC/COLLECTION: STOCKBYTE – NAME: 116086-2.PSD/PAGE: 99/CREDIT: © AMOS MORGAN/COLLECTION: PHOTODISC – NAME: SKD284372SDC_22.PSD/PAGE: 101/CREDIT: © GETTY IMAGES/STOCKDISC/COLLECTION: STOCKBYTE – NAME: LUBENOW-QUOTE.PSD/PAGE: 102/CREDIT: © MFMER – NAME: SKD245277SDC_22. PSD/PAGE: 104/CREDIT: © GETTY IMAGES/STOCKDISC/COLLECTION: STOCKBYTE – NAME: 40318.PSD/PAGE: 106/CREDIT: © KEITH BROFSKY/COLLECTION: PHOTODISC – NAME: 35011.PSD/PAGE 106/CREDIT © PHOTODISC/COLLECTION: PHOTODISC – NAME: WHITE.PSD/PAGE: 109/CREDIT: © MFMER – NAME: SNITZER.PSD/PAGE: 112/CREDIT: © MFMER – NAME: 40318.PSD/PAGE: 107/CREDIT: © KEITH BROFSKY – NAME: WEE_005R.PSD/PAGE: 114, 115/CREDIT: © EYEWIRE/COLLECTION: EYEWIRE –NAME: FAN2016254PATH.JPG/PAGE: 114/CREDIT: © MFMER – NAME: 71124.PSD/PAGE: 115/CREDIT: © STEVE MASON/COLLECTION: PHOTODISC – NAME: SOOD.PSD/PAGE: 118/CREDIT: © MFMER – NAME: E003134.PSD/PAGE: 120/CREDIT: © EYEWIRE COLLECTION/COLLECTION: PHOTODISC – NAME: OS31051.PSD/PAGE: 123/CREDIT: © C SQUARED STUDIOS/COLLECTION: C SQUARED STUDIOS – NAME: 75128.PSD/PAGE: 124/CREDIT: PHOTODISC/COLLECTION PHOTODISC – NAME: HEARTMONITOR.PSD/PAGE: 126/CREDIT: © MFMER – NAME: OS31051. PSD/PAGE: 123/CREDIT: © C SQUARED STUDIOS/COLLECTION: C SQUARED STUDIOS – NAME: HEARTCRACK.PSD/PAGE: 136/CREDIT: © MFMER – NAME: VEGGIEBACKGROUND.PSD/PAGE: 144, 145/CREDIT © MFMER - NAME: CLOGGEDPIPE.PSD/PAGE: 144/CREDIT: © MFMER – NAME: PATIENTSTORYIMAGE-UNGER.PSD/PAGE: 145/CREDIT: © MFMER – NAME: HAYES.PSD/PAGE: 151/CREDIT: © MFMER – NAME: AA050480.PSD/PAGE: 153/CREDIT: © RYAN MCVAY/COLLECTION: PHOTODISC – NAME: MCIVER.PSD/PAGE: 155/CREDIT: © MFMER – NAME: 52334.JPG/PAGE: 156/CREDIT: © STEVE COLE/COLLECTION: PHOTODISC – NAME: THOMAS-LARGE.PSD/PAGE: 156, 157/CREDIT: © MFMER – NAME: THOMAS-SMALL.PSD/PAGE: 157/CREDIT: © MFMER – NAME: STK23309WCL.PSD/PAGE: 162/CREDIT: © STOCKBYTE COLLECTION/COLLECTION: STOCKBYTE – NAME: AA051009.PSD/PAGE: 164/CREDIT: © STEVE COLE/GETTY IMAGES/COLLECTION/PHOTODISC – NAME: AA049489.PSD/PAGE: 166/CREDIT: © JIM ARBOGAST/CHAD BAKER/RYAN MCVAY/COLLECTION/PHOTODISC – NAME: PEREZ-BACKGROUND.PSD/PAGE: 166, 167/CREDIT: © MFMER – NAME: PEREZ.PSD/PAGE: 167/CREDIT: © MFMER – NAME: 484064.PSD/PAGE: 171/CREDIT: © DIGITAL VISION/COLLECTION: PHOTODISC – NAME: 8157.PSD/PAGE: 173/CREDIT: © F. SCHUSSLER/PHOTOLINK/COLLECTION/PHOTODISC – NAME: SHEN.PSD/PAGE: 172/CREDIT: © MFMER – NAME: WEF024.PSD/PAGE: 175/CREDIT: © BANANASTOCK COLLECTION/COLLECTION: BANANASTOCK – NAME: MEL_071.PSD/PAGE: 176/CREDIT: © EYEWIRE COLLECTION/COLLECTION: EYEWIRE – NAME: MAGEEBACKGROUND.PSD/PAGE: 176, 177/CREDIT: © MFMER – NAME: MAGEE.PSD/PAGE: 177/CREDIT: © MFMER – NAME: NIKOMO.PSD/PAGE: 183/CREDIT: © MFMER – NAME: 62986CORCMYK75.PSD/PAGE 185/CREDIT: © STOCKBYTE ROYALTY FREE PHOTOS/COLLECTION/PHOTODISC – NAME: 39102.PSD/PAGE: 186/CREDIT: © GEOSTOCK/COLLECTION: PHOTODISC – NAME: 16097.PSD/PAGE: 186, 187/CREDIT: © C. BORLAND/PHOTOLINK/COLLECTION PHOTODISC – NAME: KRAMER.PSD/PAGE: 187/CREDIT: © MFMER – NAME: MOUSSA-2011_14.PSD/PAGE: 193/ © MFMER – NAME: E003996R.PSD/PAGE: 192/COLLECTION - PHOTODISC – NAME: 327003RKNRGB75.PSD/PAGE: 196/CREDIT © G2-12-15-04-LSL/COLLECTION: PHOTODISC – NAME: DOCTORTRUCK.PSD/PAGE: 198, 199/CREDIT: © MFMER – NAME: DOKTOR.PSD/PAGE: 199/CREDIT © MFMER – NAME: MAGEE.PSD/PAGE: 177/CREDIT: © MFMER – NAME: NIKOMO.PSD/PAGE: 183/CREDIT: © MFMER – NAME: CONNOLLY 4.PSD/PAGE: 203/CREDIT: MFMER – NAME: AVA_012R.PSD/PAGE: 206/CREDIT: © EYEWIRE,INC./ COLLECTION: EYEWIRE, INC. – NAME: 755025.JPG/PAGE: 208/COLLECTION: PHOTODISC – NAME: 755026.JPG/PAGE: 208/COLLECTION: PHOTODISC – NAME: 18089. PSD/PAGE: 209/CREDIT: © PHOTOLINK/COLLECTION: PHOTODISC – NAME: ECA_049.PSD/PAGE: 216/CREDIT: © EYEWIRE COLLECTION/COLLECTION: EYEWIRE COLLECTION – NAME: MHE_015.PSD/PAGE: 219/COLLECTION: EYEWIRE COLLECTION – NAME: PAF090000083.JPG/PAGE: 220/CREDIT: © ISABELLE ROZENBAUM/COLLECTION: PHOTOALTO – NAME: BBA_080R.PSD/PAGE: 221/CREDIT: © EYEWIRE,INC./ COLLECTION: EYEWIRE, INC. – NAME: 48074.PSD/PAGE 224/CREDIT: © PHOTODISC/ COLLECTION: PHOTODISC – NAME: 77049.PSD/PAGE: 227/CREDIT: © NANCY R. COHEN/ COLLECTION: PHOTODISC – NAME: DV2014045.PSD/PAGE: 230/ CREDIT: © DIGITAL VISION/COLLECTION: DIGITAL VISION – NAME: PAF089000035-2.PSD/PAGE: 233 – NAME: 0611 ASIANSALMON.PSD/PAGE: 234/ CREDIT: © MFMEF – NAME: 0711 PUTTANESCARICE.PSD/PAGE: 235/CREDIT: © MFMER – NAME: GRILLEDFLANKSTEAKSALAD.PSD/PAGE: 237/CREDIT: © MFMEF – NAME: PAF089000081.PSD/PAGE: 236 – NAME: COUSCOUSSALAD.PSD/PAGE: 238/CREDIT: © MFMER – NAME: TURKEYSLOPPYJOES-2.PSD/PAGE: 239/CREDIT: © MFMER – NAME: OS1096.TIF/PAGE: 240/CREDIT: © C SQUARED STUDIOS/COLLECTION: C SQUARED STUDIOS – NAME: OS49029.PSD/PAGE: 240/CREDIT: © C SQUARED STUDIOS/COLLECTION: C SQUARED STUDIOS – NAME: 0911 APPLELETTUCESALAD_EH_RECIPE.PSD/PAGE: 241/CREDIT: © MFMER – NAME: MIXEDBERRYCOFFEECAKE.PSD/PAGE: 242/CREDIT: © MFMER – NAME: BAKEDAPPLESW_CHERRIES.EPS/PAGE: 243/CREDIT: © MFMER – NAME: 0611 ASIANSALMON.PSD/PAGE: 234 – NAME: FAN9003050. PSD/PAGE: 223/CREDIT: © MCNALYN GRAC A/CORBIS – NAME: 67183.PSD/PAGE: 227/CREDIT: © MITCH HRDLICKA/COLLECTION: PHOTODISC – NAME: OS49102.PSD/PAGE: 228/CREDIT: © C SQUARED STUDIOS/COLLECTION: PHOTODISC – NAME: PAF089000035-2.PSD/PAGE: 233/COLLECTION: PHOTOALTO – NAME: PAF090000028-2.PSD/PAGE: 231/COLLECTION: PHOTOALTO – NAME: PAF089000016-2.PSD/PAGE: 229/ CREDIT: © PHOTOALTO/COLLECTION: PHOTOALTO – NAME: 20018.PSD/PAGE: 233/CREDIT: © DENNIS GRAY/COLE GROUP/COLLECTION: PHOTODISC – NAME: 51187.JPG/PAGE: 244/CREDIT: © JACK HOLLINGSWORTH/COLLECTION: PHOTODISC – NAME: 58101.PSD/PAGE: 251/CREDIT: © STEVE MASON/COLLECTION: PHOTODISC – NAME: FAN9003010.PSD/PAGE: 247/CREDIT: © MONALYN GRACIA/CORBIS – NAME: FAN9003037.PSD/PAGE: 252/CREDIT: © MONALYN GRACIA/CORBIS/COLLECTION: CORBIS – NAME: FAN90030E0.PSD/PAGE: 249/CREDIT: © MONALYN GRACIA/CORBIS/COLLECTION: CORBIS – NAME: 116085.PSD/PAGE: 258/CREDIT: © AMOS MORGAN/COLLECTION: PHOTODISC – NAME: FAN9003106-2.PSD/PAGE: 260/CREDIT: © MONALYN GRACIA/CORBIS/COLLECTION: CORBIS – NAME: HLC073MH.PSD/PAGE: 263/CREDIT: © ARTVILLE/COLLECTION: ARTVILLE – NAME: OS1037.PSD/PAGE: 264/CREDIT: © C SQUARED STUDIOS/COLLECTION: C SQUARED STUDIOS – NAME: PAF090000062-2.PSD/PAGE: 265/CREDIT: © PHOTOALTO/COLLECTION: PHOTOALTO – NAME: 59118. PSD/PAGE: 267/CREDIT: © PHOTODISC/COLLECTION: PHOTODISC – NAME: OAD_009R.PSD/PAGE: 268/CREDIT: © EYEWIRE/COLLECTION: © EYEWIRE – NAME: 56386936_22.PSD/PAGE: 269/CREDIT: © STOCKBYTE/COLLECTION: STOCKBYTE – NAME: 32328.PSD/PAGE: 271/CREDIT: © JACK STAR/COLLECTION: PHOTOLINK – NAME: AVA_006R.PSD/PAGE: 272/CREDIT: © EYEWIRE/COLLECTION: EYEWIRE – NAME: PAF089000069.PSD/PAGE: 261 – NAME: BBA_088R.PSD/PAGE: 249/CREDIT: © EYEWIRE,INC./COLLECTION: EYEWIRE,INC. – NAME: FAN9003073.PSD/PAGE: 251/CREDIT: © MONALYN GRACIA/CORBIS – NAME: FAN9003055.PSD/PAGE: 252/CREDIT: © MONALYN GRACIA/CORBIS – NAME: BBA_021R.JPG/PAGE: 254/CREDIT: ©1998 EYEWIRE,INC./COLLECTION: EYEWIRE,INC. – NAME: OS48062.PSD/PAGE: 255/CREDIT: © SIEDE PREIS/COLLECTION: PHOTODISC

Index

A

Abdominal aortic aneurysms, 190
Acupuncture, 267
Alcohol, 173, 274, 275
Aldosterone antagonists, 165
Aneurysms, 188-190
Angicoagulants and anti-platelets, 104
Antibiotics, 204–205
Antioxidants, 262
Anxiety
  heart health link, 272–273
  self-care tips, 275
  symptoms, 275
Aorta, 188
  coarctation of, 199, 201
Aortic aneurysms
  abdominal, 190
  defined, 188–189
  family history and, 197
  screening for, 189–190
  thoracic, 190
  tobacco use and, 196
Aortic regurgitation, 178
Aortic stenosis, 178
Arrhythmias
  ablation as treatment, 172
  atrial fibrillation, 168, 169
  blood thinning medications and, 173
  bradycardia, 168, 170
  as CAD complication, 148
  caffeine or alcohol and, 173
  causes of, 168–169
  complications, 171
  as congenital heart disease complication, 202
  defined, 166
  diagnosis, 171–172
  exercise and, 173
  as heart failure cause, 159
  ICD and, 174–175
  Mayo Clinic Healthy Heart Plan for, 173–175
  over-the-counter medications and, 175
  symptoms, 170
  tachycardia, 168, 169, 170
  tobacco use and, 174
  treatment, 172–173
  as valve disorder complication, 181
  ventricular fibrillation, 170

Arthritis, 251
Aspirin, daily, 101
Atherosclerosis
  clots, 138, 139
  complications, 141
  development, 138–139
Atrial fibrillation, 168, 169
Atrial septal defect, 201
Autoimmune diseases, 85
Automatic external defibrillators (AEDs), 112-113

B

Bedtime
  eating before, 60
  physical activity and, 60–61
  routine, 60–61
Beta blockers, 104, 165
Bicuspid aortic valve (BAV), 185
Biofeedback, 266
Blood clots, 149, 150
  as aortic aneurysm complication, 190
  in atherosclerosis, 138, 139
Blood flow
  flow from heart to rest of body, 133
  oxygen exchange, 130
  to lungs, 131-132
  travel back to heart, 132
Blood pressure
  categories, 75
  diastolic, 75, 140
  in doctor's office, 216–217
  at home, 217–219
  kidneys and, 188
  measurement of, 74, 216-219
  numbers, 81
  systolic, 75, 140
  test, 73, 74
Blood sugar, 78-79
Blood tests
  cholesterol, 209
  C-reactive protein (CRP), 210
  fasting plasma glucose, 209
  fibrinogen, 210
  homocysteine, 210
  lipoprotein, 210
  natriuretic peptides, 210
  thyroid hormone, 209
Body mass index (BMI)
  body fat and, 255–256
  calculating, 73, 257

defined, 78, 255
in healthy weight, 255–256
numbers, 69, 73, 81
Bradycardia, 168, 170
Breakfast
grains at, 40
importance of, 39
time factor and, 40
tips for eating, 39–40
B-type natriuretic peptide (BNP) test, 161

C

Caffeine, 173
Calcium, as valve disorder cause, 180
Calcium channel blockers, 104
Capillaries, 135
Carbon dioxide, 132
Cardiac ablation, 172
Cardiac arrest, 111
Cardiac catheterization, 172, 215
Cardiac CT scans, 215
Cardiac MRIs, 215–216
Cardiac rehabilitation, 152
Cardiomyopathy
inheritance, 165
types of, 159
Cardiopulmonary resuscitation (CPR)
AED use and, 113
conventional, 111
defined, 110
hands-only, 111
steps, 110–111
training, 113
Cerebrovascular disease, 195
Cheese, 42
Chest pain (angina), 181
Chest X-rays, 213
Chocolate and cocoa, 265
Cholesterol, 74-75
HDL levels, 51, 76, 77
high levels as heart disease risk factor, 94
LDL levels, 50, 76, 77, 152
numbers, 81
test, 73, 75–77
total, 77
Coarctation of the aorta, 199, 201
Coenzyme Q10 (CoQ10), 262
Complementary and alternative medicine (CAM)
acupuncture, 267
benefits of, 261

biofeedback, 266
doctor consultation before, 261
food as medicine, 264–265
herbal and dietary supplements, 262–263
mind-body medicine, 266–267
using, 260–267
Computed tomography (CT), 172, 215
Congenital heart disease
antibiotics, 204–205
atrial septal defect, 201
causes, 200
coarctation of the aorta, 201
complications, 202–203
complications of surgeries, 200–201
defined, 198
diagnosis, 203–204
emergency plan, 205
exercise and, 204
family planning and, 205
genetic connection, 200
Mayo Clinic Healthy Heart Plan for, 204–205
medical history and, 204
medications, 204
misconceptions, 200
signs and symptoms, re-emergence of, 200
sleep disorders and, 205
surgery, 204
symptoms, 202
treatment, 204
types of, 200
Congestive heart failure, 143, 160–161
Continuous positive airway pressure (CPAP), 62
Coronary angioplasty procedure, 149
Coronary arteries, 129, 144, 147
Coronary artery bypass, 149, 150
Coronary artery disease (CAD)
cardiac rehabilitation and, 152
causes, identifying, 146–149
complications, 148
development, 145
diagnosis, 149
heart devices and, 153
as heart failure cause, 159
Mayo Clinic Healthy Heart Plan for, 152–153
medications and, 152–153
plaques, 146, 147
risk factors, 151
statistics, 144
symptoms, 148
treatment, 149
women and, 151

Cranberries, 264
C-reactive protein (CRP), 210
Critical limb ischemia (CLI), 192

D

Depression
    after heart event, 272
    in eating, 230
    heart health link, 272–273
    medication compliance and, 103
    recognizing, 273–274
    self-care tips, 274
    symptoms, 273
    treatment, 273–274
Diabetes
    as heart disease risk factor, 94
    as heart failure cause, 159
    risk, 79
Diastolic pressure, 140
Diet
    changing, 37
    unhealthy, as heart disease risk factor, 94
Dilated cardiomyopathy, 158, 159
Doctor
    blood pressure test in office, 216–217
    consultation before interval training, 51
    consultation before quick start, 20
    consultation before strength training, 52
    consultation before using complementary and
        alternative medicine, 261
    consultation in weight loss or quitting smoking, 70
    test results questions for, 80

E

Eat 5, Move 10, Sleep 8
    baseline for starting, 26
    defined, 27
    Eat 5, 27–28
    log or checklist, 27
    Move 10, 28–29
    Sleep 8, 29–30
Eating obstacles
    diet overhaul, 222
    meat and protein, 224
    menu planning, 226
    new foods, 225
    old recipes, 228
    overcoming, 220–243
    portion control, 231

    stress, depression and boredom, 230
    success difficulty, 232
    time for healthy meals, 221
Echocardiograms, 172
    benefits of, 213–214
    defined, 213
    for heart valve problems, 183
Ejection fraction, 142, 161
Electrical activity, heart, 130
Electrocardiograms (ECG)
    for arrhythmias, 171–172
    defined, 210
    recording, 210–211
Emergencies
    congenital heart disease and, 204–205
    CPR and, 110–111, 113
    delay and, 109–110
    family involvement in, 113
    heart attack, 108
    heart failure, 108–109
    high blood pressure, 108
    planning for, 106–113
    valve disorders as, 180
Enjoying life
    adaptability and, 120–121
    appreciation, 116–117
    benefits of, 115
    keys to, 116–121
    laughing, 117
    leisure time, 117
    listening, 117
    online social networking, 116
    pets, 117
    realistic balance, 121
    relaxation, 115
    relaxation techniques, 117
    social network support, 113
    stress and, 118–120
    support, 117
    volunteering, 116
Erectile dysfunction (ED), 194
Exercise. See Physical activity
Exercise obstacles
    appearance, 249
    don't like it, 247
    expense, 250
    overcoming, 244–253
    pain, 251
    time, 245
    too tired, 246
    weather, 248

Exercise stress test, 212
Expectations, Mayo Clinic Healthy Heart Plan, 22–23

F

Familial hyperlipidemia (FH), 76
Family history
  adoption and, 87
  collecting, 87
  confidentiality, 87
  as heart disease risk factor, 86, 94
  indicating factors, 87
  inheritance, 85
  medical trees, 87, 88
  questions, 87–88
  vascular disorders and, 197
Family planning, 205
Family screening
  heart failure, 165
  heart valve disorders, 185
Fats
  monounsaturated, 41
  reduced, products, 42
  saturated, 41
  trimming from meat, 43
  unhealthy, reducing, 42
Fibrinogen, 210
Fish, 42, 43, 264
Flaxseed oil, 262
Fluid intake, 163
Food as medicine, 264–265

G

Garlic, 262–263
Ginkgo, 262–263
Ginseng, 262–263
Goals
  charting, 123
  do's and don'ts of setting, 97
  Eat 5, Move 10, Sleep 8, 27
  enjoying life, 115
  healthy diet, 37
  lapses, dealing with, 120
  medications, 99
  numbers, 73
  outcome, 91
  performance, 91
  quick start scorecard, 30
  sleep, 57
  smoking cessation, 65

targets, 91
weight loss, 65
working towards, 121
Grains
  sticky, 265
  tips for eating, 40–41
Grapes (including wine), 264–265

H

Hawthorn, 262–263
Healthy diet
  balance principle, 44
  breakfast, 39–40
  DASH diet, 223
  fats and, 41–42
  fruits and vegetables, 38–39
  goals, 37
  grains, 40–41
  guide to, 36–45
  keys to, 38
  Mayo Clinic Diet, 222
  Mediterranean diet, 223
  moderation principle, 44
  MyPlate, 45
  protein, 42–43, 224
  salt and, 41
  serving sizes, 45
  tips for living, 44
  variety principle, 44
Healthy eating
  on busy schedule, 221
  with family, 225
  foods to have on hand, 226
  fullness feeling, 231
  with heart-healthy eating plan, 222
  moods and, 230
  nutritional labels and, 227
  obstacles, overcoming, 220–243
  portion size, 231
  recipe adaptation chart, 229
  recipe transformation, 228
  recipes, 234–243
  success, 232
Healthy weight
  benefits of, 254
  body mass index (BMI), 255–256
  defined, 255
  finding, 254–259
  personal medical history, 256–258
  waist measurement, 256

Heart
    in blood circulation, 127
    chambers, 128
    coronary arteries, 129, 144, 147
    diastole, 140
    with dilated cardiomyopathy, 158
    ejection fraction, 142, 161
    electrical activity, 130
    functioning of, 126–143
    high blood pressure and, 140
    with hypertrophic cardiomyopathy, 158
    speeding up or slowing down medications, 173
    statistics, 126
    stress and, 269
    systole, 140
    valves, 128
Heart attack
    as CAD complication, 148
    chances, 93
    as medical emergency, 108, 137
    prevention, 150
    sudden cardiac arrest versus, 111
    survival plan, 113
    uncommon causes of, 146
Heart disease
    aspirin and, 101
    sleep and obesity and, 61
    sleep apnea and, 62
Heart disease risk
    calculators, 93
    clues to, 84
    family history and, 86
    personal factors, 92
    women's, 85
Heart failure
    as arrhythmia complication, 171
    as CAD complication, 148
    causes, 159
    as congenital heart disease complication, 203
    congestive, 143, 160–161
    defined, 156
    diagnosis, 161
    diet changes and, 17
    emergencies, 108–109
    exercise and, 163–164
    family screening, 165
    fluid intake and, 163
    ICD and, 165
    Mayo Clinic Healthy Heart Plan for, 162–165
    potassium and, 164
    salt and, 162

    sleep disorders and, 164
    symptoms, 160
    treatment, 161
    as valve disorder complication, 181
    weight gain and, 162–163
Heart health
    depression or anxiety and, 272–273
    ejection fraction and, 142
    lifestyle impact on, 115
    numbers for, 74–79
    physical activity and, 48
    tobacco and, 66-67
    weight and, 68-69
Heart medications, 104
Heart murmurs, 182
Heart valve disorders
    aortic regurgitation, 178
    aortic stenosis, 178
    causes, 178–181
    complications, 181
    as congenital heart disease complication, 203
    dental work and, 184–185
    diagnosis, 182
    as emergencies, 180
    exercise and, 184
    family screening, 185
    leaflets, 176
    Mayo Clinic Healthy Heart Plan for, 184–185
    medications and, 182
    mitral prolapse, 179
    mitral regurgitation, 178, 179
    mitral stenosis, 178
    symptoms, 181
    treatment, 182–183
    types of, 178
Herbal and dietary supplements
    antioxidants, 262
    herbs, 262–263
    oils, 262
    red yeast rice, 263
    reading label before taking, 263
    vitamin D, 263
High blood pressure
    complications, 141
    defined, 188
    emergencies, 108
    heart and, 140
    as heart disease risk factor, 94
    as heart failure cause, 159
    pulmonary hypertension, 188
    weight training and, 253

High-density lipoprotein (HDL), 51, 76, 77
History
    congenital heart disease and, 204
    family, 85–88
    in healthy weight, 256–258
    personal, 83–84
    women's unique risks and, 85
Home blood pressure monitoring, 217-219
    radial pulse, 219
Homocysteine, 210
Hypertrophic cardiomyopathy, 158, 159

Imaging tests
    cardiac catheterization, 215
    cardiac CT scans, 215
    cardiac MRIs, 215–216
    chest X-ray, 213
    echocardiogram, 213–214
    transesophageal ultrasound, 214
Implantable cardioverter-defibrillator (ICD), 153, 161, 165, 174–175
Infections
    as congenital heart disease complication, 202
    as valve disorder cause, 180
    as valve disorder complication, 181
Interval training 50-51

K

Kidneys, in blood pressure control, 188

L

Lapses, dealing with, 120
Low-density lipoprotein (LDL), 50, 76, 77, 152
Lungs, 131-132
    oxygen exchange, 132
    problems as valve disorder complication, 181

M

Magnetic resonance imaging (MRI), 172, 182, 215–216
Marfan syndrome, 190, 197
Mayo Clinic Diet, 222
Mayo Clinic Healthy Heart Plan
    for arrhythmias, 173–175
    for CAD, 152–153
    for congenital heart disease, 204–205

    doctor consultation before starting, 20
    eat healthy, 35, 36–45
    emergencies, 35, 106–113
    enjoy life, 35, 114–123
    for heart failure, 162–165
    for heart valve disorders, 184–185
    history, 35, 82–89
    medications, 35, 98–105
    numbers, 35, 72–81
    physical activity, 35, 46
    sleep, 35, 56–63
    smoking, 35, 64–71
    steps for starting, 21
    targets, 35, 90–97
    for vascular disease, 196–197
    weight, 35, 64–71
Mayo Clinic Healthy Weight Pyramid, 69, 222, 259
Meat
    in healthy diet, 224
    in recipe adaptation, 229
    trimming fat from, 43
Medication side effects, 104-105
    challenges, overcoming, 102
    statin, 105
Medications
    aldosterone antagonists, 165
    angicoagulants and anti-platelets, 104
    angiotensin-converting enzyme (ACE) inhibitors, 104
    aspirin, 101
    beta blockers, 104, 165
    blood thinning, 173
    CAD and, 152–153
    calcium channel blockers, 104
    challenges, overcoming, 102–103
    congenital heart disease, 204
    depression and, 103
    digoxin, 165
    heart, 104
    heart valve disorders and, 182
    nitrates, 104
    problem, understanding, 100
    questions about, 100
    remembering challenge, 102
    routine change challenge, 103
    for speeding up or slowing down heart, 173
    statins, 104, 105
    too expensive challenge, 103
    too many challenge, 103
    uncertainty challenge, 103
    vasodilators, 165
    water pills (diuretics), 104, 165

Meditation, 267
Mediterranean diet, 223
Mental health
    anxiety, 275
    depression, 272–274
    monitoring, 268–275
    stress, 269–271
Metabolic syndrome, 80
Mind-body medicine, 266–267
Mitral regurgitation, 179
Mitral stenosis, 178
Mitral valve prolapse, 179
Motivation, 20-21
    activity selection and, 52–53
    in smoking cessation, 70
    in weight loss, 70
Myocarditis, 159
MyPlate, 45

N

Naps, 61
Natriuretic peptides, 210
Nitrates, 104
Nonexercise stress test, 212–213
Numbers
    blood pressure, 74
    blood sugar, 78–79
    body mass index (BMI), 69, 78, 81
    cholesterol, 74–77
    at a glance, 81
    for heart health, 74–79
    metabolic syndrome, 80
    questions for your doctor, 80
    target, 95
    triglycerides, 77
Nutritional labels, 227
Nuts, 42, 43, 265

O

Obesity
    as heart disease risk factor, 94
    medical risks, 68
    sleep and, 61
Olive oil, 264
Omega-3 fatty acids, 262
Oral contraceptive use, 85
Outcome goals
    defined, 91
    as targets, 95

P

Performance goals
    defined, 91
    progress, tracking, 96
Peripheral arterial disease (PAD)
    defined, 191
    diagnostic test for, 193
    family history and, 197
    feet protection and, 197
    screening for, 192–193
    symptoms of, 191–192
    tobacco use and, 196
    walking for, 193–195
Personal medical history
    building, 83–84
    in healthy weight, 256–258
Physical activity
    activity selection, 52–53
    anxiety and, 275
    appearance while engaging, 249
    arrhythmias and, 173
    arthritis and, 251
    congenital heart disease and, 204
    cost, minimizing, 250
    depression and, 274
    enjoyable, making, 247
    finding time for, 245
    heart failure and, 163–164
    heart health and, 48
    heart valve disorders and, 184
    incorporation into day, 246
    increasing, 48
    interval training, 50–51
    lack of, as heart disease risk factor, 94
    low impact, 252
    modification strategies, 252–253
    Move 10, 28–29
    official recommendations, 28
    safety, 252
    with "stealing time," 48
    strength training, 52
    as stress buster, 51
    types of, 29
    warming up before, 50
    weather options, 248
    weight training, 252–253
Plant sterols or stanols, 264
Plaques, 138, 139, 146, 147
Postmenopausal hormone therapy, 85
Potassium, 164
Prediabetes, 79

Pregnancy complications, 85
Progressive relaxation, 266–267
Protein, 42-43
  strategies, 224
Pulmonary hypertension, 188, 203

Q

Qi gong, 267
Quick start, 24-31
  assessment, 22-23
  doctor consultation before beginning, 20
  Eat 5, Move 10, Sleep 8, 27–30
  motivation for, 20-21
  progress, tracking, 25
  scorecard, 30

R

Radial pulse, taking, 219
Recipes
  adaptation chart, 229
  Apple Lettuce Salad, 241
  Baked Apples with Cherries and Almonds, 243
  Chicken Stir-Fry with Eggplant and Basil, 236
  Couscous Salad, 238
  Grilled Asian Salmon, 234
  Grilled Flank Steak Salad, 237
  Minestrone Soup, 240
  Mixed Berry Whole-Grain Coffee Cake, 242
  Puttanesca with Brown Rice, 235
  Springtime Pea Soup, 240
  10-minute ideas, 233
  transforming for healthy eating, 228
  Turkey Veggie Sloppy Joes, 239
Red yeast rice, 263
Regurgitation, 178
Relaxation techniques, 117, 275
Restrictive cardiomyopathy, 159
Rheumatic fever, as valve disorder cause, 180
Risk calculators, 93

S

Salt, 17, 41, 162
Sarcoidosis, 157
Sedentary time, reducing, 49
Servings
  fruits and vegetables, 26
  sizes, 26, 45
Sex, vascular health and, 194

Sleep
  alcohol and, 61
  anxiety and, 275
  bedtime routine, 29, 60–61
  benefits of, 56
  caffeine and, 61
  congenital heart disease and, 204–205
  depression and, 274
  deprivation, 57
  diary, 63
  disorders, 61–62
  environment, 60
  general guideline, 29
  heart failure and, 164
  keys to, 58–62
  naps and, 61
  obesity and, 61
  problems, as heart disease risk factor, 94
  Sleep 8, 29–30
  slumber number, 58, 59
  tips for, 58–59
  weight loss and, 59
Sleep apnea, 61, 62
Slumber number, 58, 59
Smoking
  arrhythmias and, 174
  bodily effects of, 66
  as heart disease risk factor, 94
  as leading preventable cause of death, 66
Smoking cessation
  benefits of, 67
  medications, 67
  readiness for, 70
  resources, 66
  strategies for starting, 70–71
  support for, 70–71
  weight loss link, 65
Soybeans, 265
Statins, 104, 105
Stenosis, 178
Strength training
  benefits of, 51
  tips for, 52
Stress
  arrhythmias and, 175
  causes (stressors), 118–119, 270
  in eating, 230
  exercise and, 51
  heart and, 269
  as heart disease risk factor, 94
  recognizing, 119

Stress management
    in enjoying life, 118–120
    importance of, 269
    stressor identification for, 270
    for weight loss or quitting smoking, 70–71
Stress tests
    defined, 211
    exercise, 212
    nonexercise, 212–213
Stroke
    as arrhythmia complication, 171
    as congenital heart disease complication, 202
    signs and symptoms, 195
Sudden cardiac death, 171
Support, 70-71, 117
Systolic pressure, 140

T

Tachycardia, 168, 169, 170
Tai Chi, 267
Targets
    goals, 91
    numbers, 95
    outcome goals as, 95
    performance goals and, 96
    plans to reach, 95–96
Tea and coffee, 265
Tests
    blood, 209–210
    blood pressure, 74, 216–219
    blood sugar, 78–79
    blood tests, 209–210
    diagnostic, 208–219
    electrocardiogram, 210–211
    imaging, 213–216
    stress, 211–213
    stress tests, 211–213
    triglycerides, 77
    walk-in heart scans, 214
Thoracic aortic aneurysms, 190
Transesophageal ultrasound, 214
Triglycerides, 77, 81

V

Vascular disorders
    cerebrovascular disease, 195
    diseases of the aorta, 188
    exercise and, 196
    family history and, 197

high-blood pressure, 188
    Mayo Clinic Healthy Heart Plan for, 196–197
    peripheral arterial disease (PAD), 191–195
    sex and, 194
    tobacco use and, 196
    walking program and, 196–197
Vasodilators, 165
Vegetables and fruit
    Eat 5 goal, 27–28
    increasing intake of, 38–39
Ventricular fibrillation, 170
Vitamins C, D and E, 262-263

W

Waist measurement
    fat distribution and, 256
    importance of, 78
    numbers, 78, 256
Walk-in heart scans, warning, 214
Walking
    benefits, 29
    in interval training, 51
    for PAD, 193–195
    personal safety, 55
    routes, 55
    12-week schedule, 54
Water pills (diuretics), 104, 165
Weight
    heart health and, 68–69
    ideal, 258
Weight gain, 162–163
Weight loss
    benefits of, 68–69
    goals, 65
    resources, 68
    sleep and, 58
    smoking link, 65
    strategies for starting, 70–71
    stress management, 71
Weight training
    caution with, 252–253
    high blood pressure and, 253
Women
    autoimmune conditions, 151
    CAD and, 151
    risks, 85

Y

Yoga, 267

You can seek the help of one doctor.

Or you can turn to Mayo Clinic.

At Mayo Clinic, a team of experts works together for you. No wonder Mayo Clinic's collective knowledge and innovative treatments have been a shining light to millions around the world. Visit mayoclinic.org/connect to learn from others who've been there.

Did you know that anyone can request an appointment at Mayo Clinic? If a physician referral is required, our appointment staff will advise you. All appointments are prioritized on the basis of medical need and are scheduled as early as possible. Please call 507-266-6160 to schedule an appointment.

MAYO
CLINIC

PHOENIX/SCOTTSDALE, ARIZONA | ROCHESTER, MINNESOTA | JACKSONVILLE, FLORIDA

Visit our online store

for a wide selection of books, newsletters and DVDs developed by Mayo Clinic doctors and editorial staff.

Discover practical, easy-to-understand information on topics of interest to millions of health-conscious people like you ...

➤ *Mayo Clinic Health Letter* — our award-winning monthly newsletter filled with practical information on today's health and medical news

➤ *Mayo Clinic Family Health Book* — the ultimate home health reference

➤ *The Mayo Clinic Diet: Eat Well, Enjoy Life, Lose Weight* — step-by-step guidance from Mayo Clinic weight-loss experts to help you achieve a healthy weight.

➤ *Mayo Clinic Book of Alternative Medicine* — the new approach to combining the best of natural therapies and conventional medicine

➤ *Mayo Clinic Book of Home Remedies* — discover how to prevent, treat or manage over 120 common health conditions at home

➤ *Mayo Clinic on Digestive Health* — learn how to identify and treat digestive problems before they become difficult to manage

➤ *Plus* — books on arthritis, aging, diabetes, high blood pressure and other conditions

Mayo Clinic brings you more of the health information you're looking for!

Learn more at:

www.Store.MayoClinic.com

U.S., Canada and International order processing available.